THE COMPLETE GUIDE TO
AQUA EXERCISE FOR PREGNANCY AND POSTNATAL HEALTH

Sarah Bolitho and Vicky Hatch

B L O O M S B U R Y

LONDON • NEW DELHI • NEW YORK • SYDNEY

Note

While every effort has been made to ensure that the content of this book is as technically accurate and as sound as possible, neither the author nor the publishers can accept responsibility for any injury or loss sustained as a result of the use of this material.

Published by Bloomsbury Publishing Plc
50 Bedford Square
London WC1B 3DP
www.bloomsbury.com

First edition 2014
Copyright © 2014 Sarah Bolitho and Vicky Hatch
ISBN (print): 978-1-4081-9274-0
ISBN (epub): 978-1-4081-9275-7
ISBN (epdf): 978-1-4081-9276-4

A CIP catalogue record for this book is available from the British Library.

Acknowledgements
Cover photograph © Getty Images
All images © Shutterstock with the exception of the following; pp. viii, 45, 54, 56 and 62 © Getty Images
Illustrations by Dave Gardner
Commissioning Editor: Charlotte Croft
Editor: Sarah Cole
Designer: James Watson

This book is produced using paper that is made from wood grown in managed, sustainable forests. It is natural, renewable and recyclable. The logging and manufacturing processes conform to the environmental regulations of the country of origin.

Typeset in 10.75pt on 14pt Adobe Caslon by seagulls.net

Printed and bound in China by Leo Paper Products

10 9 8 7 6 5 4 3 2 1

THE COMPLETE GUIDE TO
AQUA EXERCISE FOR PREGNANCY AND POSTNATAL HEALTH

CONTENTS

INTRODUCTION

The aim of this book is to review the benefits of water-based exercise during pregnancy and the postnatal period to provide a unique reference guide for fitness instructors or midwives who may be involved in prescribing exercise programmes for pre- or postnatal women. It is also suitable for aqua instructors who may encounter occasional pre- or postnatal women within their water-based activity sessions, or aqua instructors whose class participants become pregnant.

We hope this book will be a complete resource for any practitioner working with pre- and post-natal women in water. It is designed to support the National Occupational Standards for the Level 2 Certificate in Fitness Instructing (Water-Based Exercise) and the Level 3 Award in Adapting Activity for Antenatal and Postnatal Clients, and combines the knowledge of these two fitness modes. The inclusion of an extensive range of exercises and class formats makes this a valuable, user-friendly resource that can be referred to on an ongoing basis for information and ideas.

We recommend that anyone who intends to deliver aqua-natal sessions is either already qualified or undertakes a specific training course such as the Level 3 Award in Adapting Activity for Antenatal and Postnatal Clients, and the Level 2 Certificate in Fitness Instructing (Water-Based Exercise), both of which cover the relevant underpinning knowledge in more depth. Midwives who want to deliver water-based exercise to their patients are advised to work alongside a qualified

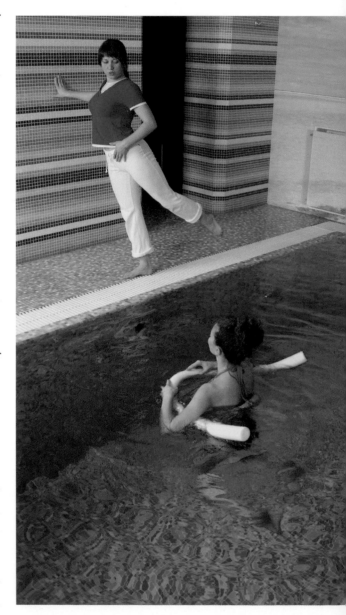

instructor or to gain the Level 2 Certificate in Fitness Instructing (Water-Based Exercise).

Aquatic training, or water-based exercise, is one of the most accessible exercise disciplines and can be adapted for all levels of fitness and ability. The resistance of the water supports the body and requires exercises to be performed at a slower speed, which makes water-based exercise sessions attractive and safe not only for those who are pregnant but also for beginners, older participants and for people carrying additional bodyweight.

Regular exercisers and non-exercising women may try water-based activity during pregnancy in order to stay healthy and mobile and to try to relieve some of the discomforts of pregnancy. Offering aqua-natal sessions means midwives, fitness instructors and swimming teachers who hold appropriate qualifications can support women with a 'normal' pregnancy who want to take up or maintain activity. As well as helping to manage any aches or pains they might be experiencing, this will also provide a wealth of health-related benefits for both mother and baby.

It is normal for a pregnant woman to be concerned about exercising and the potential risks to the pregnancy and her baby. However, research now suggests that moderate exercise, particularly exercise in water, is safe and may even be beneficial for maternal health and foetal outcome (Katz, 1996; Kihlstrand et al, 1999; Hartmann & Bung, 1999; Clapp, 2000; Lox, 2000; Parker & Smith, 2003; Smith & Michel, 2006; and 2003; NICE, 2007), thus more women may seek opportunities to participate in this type of activity during pregnancy.

Acknowledgements

Sarah Bolitho
Thanks and gratitude to Vicky Hatch for working with me on this book. It is always a pleasure and a learning journey when we work together. Thank you also to everyone at Bloomsbury for giving me another chance to put my passion for writing into action.

Vicky Hatch
Thanks to Sarah Bolitho for suggesting the idea of this book and for her positive and invaluable feedback which guided every stage of our writing together.

Gratitude also goes to my husband, Chris, for his unwavering support and for doing the ironing.

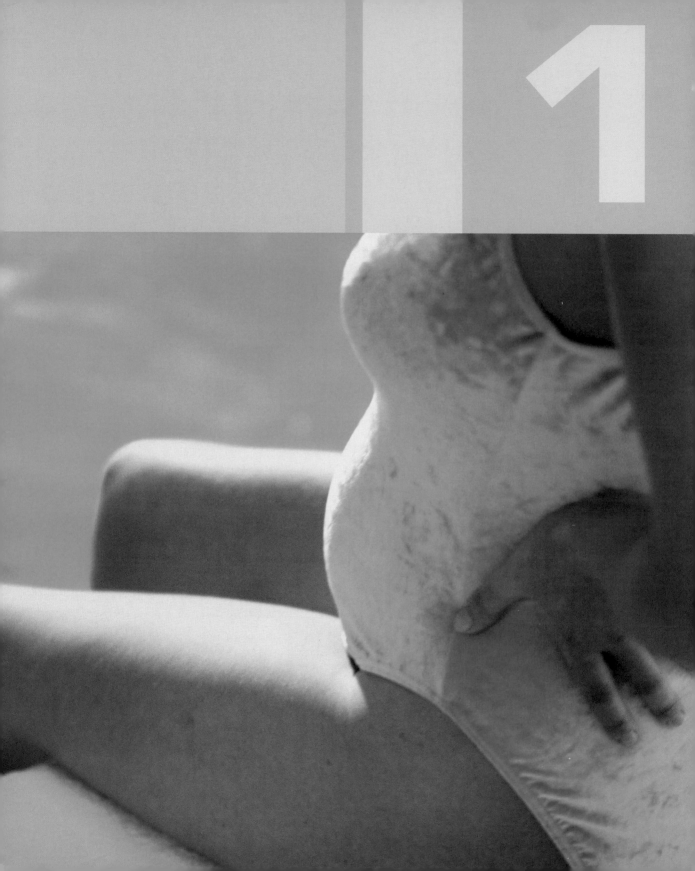

PART **ONE**

UNDERPINNING KNOWLEDGE

This section covers the underpinning knowledge that will help you to plan and deliver safe and effective water-based sessions for pregnant and postnatal women. Chapter 1 reviews the benefits of exercise in pregnancy and looks at current levels of women who are active, both generally and during pregnancy. Chapter 2 reviews the key anatomical and physiological changes of pregnancy and the postnatal period relevant to water-based exercise including cardiovascular, respiratory and musculoskeletal implications. Chapter 3 considers the properties of water and how physiological changes, including increases in weight and body mass in pregnancy, affect participation in water-based exercise. Chapter 4 looks at the benefits of water-based exercise in pregnancy and the postnatal period, and also covers the risks and contraindications to activity at this time.

ACTIVITY IN PREGNANCY

OVERVIEW OF ACTIVITY LEVELS IN PREGNANT WOMEN

It is a fact that the majority of women in the UK are inactive with only 29 per cent self-reporting that they meet the current recommendations for activity for health (see Appendix 1). When accelerometers, devices that measure movement accurately, were used to measure activity, the figure dropped to around 4 per cent of women who were active enough to gain health benefits. The figures for pregnant women are equally low, as only 23 per cent self-report being active at or above the recommended levels in the past month. This low level of activity may be linked to the rising levels of obesity and being overweight in adult women in the UK; currently an estimated 32 per cent of women are classified as overweight and 26.1 per cent as obese – meaning around 58 per cent of adult women in the UK are over the recommended weight guidelines (Public Health England, UK Prevalance and Trends, 2013).

PREGNANCY AND OBESITY

Just as with women in general, rates of being overweight or obese in women of childbearing age are rising. Nearly half of women of childbearing age in the UK are overweight or obese, with an estimated 22 per cent obese and, as maternal obesity carries significant risks for both maternal and foetal health, this is a major concern. Women may be overweight or obese prior to becoming pregnant, or may gain excess weight during pregnancy ('eating for two'). Whichever is the case, excess maternal weight may linger after delivery and might not be lost before the next pregnancy, during which more weight may be gained, and not lost, creating a cycle of pregnancy and weight gain.

While avoidance of obesity is not the only reason for being active during pregnancy, it is a key one as not only are the risks of pregnancy complications increased, but also the risk of morbidity and mortality of both mother and foetus/baby when maternal obesity exists. In fact, the UK Confidential Enquiry into Maternal and Child Health (CEMACH, 2007) identifies obesity as the fastest growing cause of women dying in pregnancy or childbirth in the UK. Information available shows that more than half of deaths from indirect or direct causes in pregnancy were in women who were overweight or obese, with 15 per cent having a BMI of greater than 40.

PATTERNS AND DETERMINANTS OF ACTIVITY IN PREGNANCY

With fewer than 30 per cent of adult women meeting the activity guidelines for health, it is perhaps not surprising that activity levels in pregnant women are also low. Moreover, participation in activity on a regular basis was particularly low (Gaston & Cramp, 2011; Haakstad et al, 2009). Research indicates that while over half of the pregnant women surveyed stated that they had done moderate to vigorous household or leisure activity in the past month, fewer than 25 per cent actually met the guidelines for activity throughout their pregnancy (Evenson & Wen, 2010). Rates of activity post-partum are also low, with less than one-third of women meeting the guidelines (Durham et al, 2011). It is also indicated that activity levels tend to be much higher in the first trimester than in the second or third trimesters and that women from a white ethnic group are more likely to be active than those from other ethnic backgrounds. Add in the fact that over 15 per cent were watching over five hours of television a day and risks from inactivity start to add up.

A review of patterns and determinants of exercise during pregnancy (Gaston & Cramp, 2011) indicates that pregnant women are generally less active than non-pregnant women and that physical activity decreases during pregnancy. Predictors of higher exercise participation were being previously active, being from a white ethnic group, pregnant with their first child, and higher income and education levels. The Danish National Birth Cohort (Juhl et al, 2012) indicates that regular exercise participation during pregnancy is linked to a number of correlates, i.e. things that have an effect on or depend on another variable. Older age, being a student or unemployed, eating a healthy diet, moderate alcohol consumption and eating disorders were correlated with exercising more than three times per week. On the other hand, multiparity (carrying two or more foetuses, or in a second or subsequent pregnancy), normal or lower rated health, smoking and a poor diet were the strongest predictors of not exercising. Interestingly women aged over 25 who had metabolic or psychiatric disorders or had received fertility treatment were more likely to show increased activity levels from early to late pregnancy.

As has been discussed, activity is relatively low in pregnancy and appears to peak in the first trimester, reducing in second and third trimesters. Activity patterns pre-pregnancy appear to be linked to ongoing activity during pregnancy (Haakstad et al, 2009) and those women who were overweight or obese before pregnancy were less likely to be active during pregnancy, with less than 11 per cent of women defined as regular exercisers by the third trimester. This fall in activity levels was linked to high weight gain during pregnancy as well as being overweight or obese prior to conception. Another study found that prior to pregnancy around 46 per cent of women were active but this reduced to 28 per cent in week 17 and just over 20 per cent by the thirtieth week. However, the number of women swimming actually increased up to the thirtieth week of pregnancy (Owe et al, 2009).

It may be that pregnancy in itself is an event that leads to decreased participation in physical activity as most women reduce their activity in the first 20 weeks (Fell et al, 2009). This may be an issue that can be addressed within health care provision, since research indicates that there is little awareness among pregnant women of the benefits of activity for the baby and midwives are ideally placed to provide this information (Weir et al, 2010). Furthermore, a survey carried out jointly by the Royal College of Midwives and NetMums in 2010 found that nearly two-thirds of women (61 per cent) felt that their midwife did not have time to talk about weight management, so perhaps one of the barriers to activity is a lack of informed and trusted information and advice. A safe, effective and enjoyable aqua-natal session, run by a trained health care or fitness professional, is an ideal forum for education about starting or maintaining an active and healthy pregnancy.

KEY BENEFITS OF ACTIVITY IN PREGNANCY

There are many benefits in being active for all women, and these are just as important, if not more so, for pregnant women. The benefits of regular exercise and daily physical activity are well documented and include improved cardio-vascular fitness, muscular strength and endurance, maintenance or improvement of bone mineral density, better posture, reduced backache or back-pain, weight maintenance, mental health benefits, better ability to cope with stress, reduced risk factors for certain diseases and better management of medical conditions. There are additional bene-fits for both mother and baby to be gained from being active in pregnancy. These are discussed further in Chapter 2 and include:

- Better pregnancy posture
- Increased self-confidence
- Better circulation
- Maintenance of bone density
- Social aspect
- Control of weight gain
- Reduced pregnancy-associated long-term memory impairment
- Quicker postnatal recovery
- Less fat on baby
- Improved ability to cope with the stress of delivery (baby and mother)
- Improved ability to self-soothe (baby)

PREGNANCY AND THE IMPLICATIONS FOR AQUA EXERCISE

2

THE TIMELINE OF PREGNANCY

The following overview of the timeline of pregnancy shows the effects on the body during each trimester.

Table 2.1	The pregnancy timeline
Trimester one	
Conception	
Missed period	Often the first sign, but with increased accuracy of tests, pregnancy may be detected before a period is missed
Nausea/sickness	So called 'morning' sickness may make an unwelcome appearance and sense of taste and smell may alter
Breast tenderness	Breasts may be tender or painful within a couple of weeks of conception so a good bra is essential even at this stage
Urination	Hormones and relaxation of smooth muscle tissue in the bladder can cause increased frequency of urination
Tiredness and fainting	The many changes occurring in the body can cause dizziness, tiredness and fatigue
Joints	Relaxin is being released so joints may start to feel unstable
Mood	Fluctuating hormone levels can cause mood swings and this can be an anxious time while parents wait for the first scan

Table 2.1	The pregnancy timeline (cont.)
Trimester two	
Nausea	This will diminish in most women around 13–16 weeks, but may continue longer for some
Mood	Feelings of well-being and good health are common now
Joints	Instability may affect balance and range of movement and the larger abdomen may cause lordosis leading to backache
Supine hypotensive syndrome	When lying on the back the weight of the uterus can cause pressure on the vena cava compromising venous return to the heart, causing dizziness or nausea
The abdomen	As the foetus grows the uterus expands out of the pelvis and into the abdominal cavity
Breathing	Breathlessness is likely at this stage
Trimester three	
The abdomen	Now much larger, making breathing, eating and sleeping uncomfortable and making some movements awkward
Tiredness	This may be increasing as the body becomes heavier and may affect everyday activities
Balance	Balance may be affected by the change in centre of gravity
Joints	Unstable joints and poor posture can lead to aches and pains
Oedema	Fluid retention causes swelling, usually in wrists, hands and ankles
Breathing	The reduced space for the lungs causes breathlessness
Urination	By the end of trimester three the bladder will be under pressure from the foetus, making urination more frequent and urgent
Alertness	The so-called 'baby brain' may be evident now!
Anxiety	Fear of delivery and worry about looking after a new baby may cause anxiety
Breasts	Likely to be heavy, tender and possibly leaking milk

THE PHYSIOLOGICAL EFFECTS OF PREGNANCY

This section provides a brief summary of the key effects of pregnancy on the body. It is not intended to provide a comprehensive review of how pregnancy affects physiology; for instructors who want to understand the effects of pregnancy on the body and mind we recommend further reading or training to support this book.

Table 2.2	Overview of the key effects of pregnancy		
System	**1st trimester**	**2nd trimester**	**3rd trimester**
Cardiovascular	• Increase in resting heart rate (about 5–10 bpm) • Increase in blood volume starts • Vascular underfill may occur	• Venous return impaired causing dizziness • Blood volume now stabilised and blood pressure returns to normal	• Possible gestational hypertension • Risk of pre-eclampsia
Respiratory	• More sensitive to carbon dioxide • Increase in breathing rate • Tiredness and breathlessness may occur with any increases in activity	• Reduced space for lung expansion may lead to breathlessness with normal activity levels	• Breathing shallow due to limited space for lung expansion • Breathlessness may occur at low levels of exertion
Musculoskeletal	• The hormone relaxin is released which allows ligaments to stretch	• Increased kyphotic posture due to weight of breasts • Increased lumbar lordosis • Backache is common due to postural changes	• Effects of relaxin are at a peak now • Posture continues to be a problem and can exacerbate existing problems • Pelvis may become unstable • Pelvic girdle pain may occur
Urinary	• Hormones and increased progesterone can cause increased micturition (urination) and inability to fully empty bladder • Risk of urinary tract infection (UTI) due to incomplete emptying	• Pressure on pelvic floor can lead to incontinence	• Increased need to urinate can occur due to pressure on the bladder

Table 2.2	Overview of the key effects of pregnancy (cont.)		
Metabolic	• Increase in metabolic rate • Average healthy weight gain is 1–3 kg • No need for extra calories yet	• Risk of gestational diabetes • Average healthy weight gain is 6–8 kg • Need additional 300 kcal per day	• Risk of gestational diabetes • Average healthy weight gain is about 3–4 kg • Keep to 300 kcal per day extra intake
Gastrointestinal	• Nausea and sickness often occur • The intestinal tract relaxes	• Indigestion and heartburn common	• Constipation, indigestion and heartburn common • Piles may develop
Other	• Body temperature increases • The breasts and the uterus start to enlarge	• Hormones stabilise • Bleeding gums • A dark vertical line on the abdomen (linea negra) appears • Reactions slower	• Braxton Hicks contractions felt • Breasts enlarge and may leak • Sleep may be disrupted • Carpal tunnel syndrome • Swelling common (oedema) • Leg cramps can occur
Psychological	• Anxiety	• Mood improves	• Anxiety • Fear of birth

THE ENDOCRINE SYSTEM AND HORMONES OF PREGNANCY

There are a range of hormones that have specific effects on the body during pregnancy. The three key ones are oestrogen, progesterone and relaxin.

Oestrogen

Oestrogen is always present in women and men, although women have much higher levels. During pregnancy, oestrogen levels rise by 20–30 times, as its key function is to promote growth of the baby. It also promotes growth of the uterus, which increases about 20 times in size from the size of a fist to the size of a large watermelon.

Additional effects are on the breasts which grow to facilitate milk production, and the heart which enlarges to cope with the additional demands of pregnancy. Another effect of oestrogen is on tissue growth and this can lead to fluid retention and oedema (swelling).

Progesterone

During pregnancy, blood volume increases by up to 50 per cent to cope with the demands of the body and the growing foetus. One of the most important effects of progesterone in pregnancy is to relax smooth muscle tissue to cope with this extra volume and prevent hypertension. However,

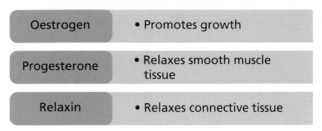

Figure 2.1 Key hormones of pregnancy

this effect is not limited to the vascular system but also affects the gastrointestinal system and urinary systems leading to possible constipation, piles, indigestion and heartburn as well as causing bladder urgency or incomplete emptying. A further effect is to raise the body's basal temperature by about 0.5–0.6 degrees Celsius during the first 20 weeks of pregnancy which can make women feel uncomfortably warm, both generally and particularly during any physical activity.

Relaxin

Relaxin is produced by the ovaries in the first trimester after which production switches to the placenta. Its function is to relax connective tissue to allow the pelvis to widen and facilitate childbirth. However, its action is not limited to the pelvis and it affects connective tissue in all joints, making them hypermobile and potentially unstable.

Relaxin is released throughout pregnancy but has the greatest effect in the third trimester. Production ceases with delivery, nevertheless the effects can remain for several months postnatally, particularly if breastfeeding. Relaxin levels in second or multiple gestation (multipara) pregnancies are higher which means additional care should be taken to protect the joints.

Other effects of relaxin include a reduction in blood clotting, inhibition of histamine release, a reduction in uterine activity and preparation (or ripening) of the cervix.

Other hormones of pregnancy

There are several other hormones that are active in pregnancy and we have included brief information below of the ones you should be aware of.

Human chorionic gonadotropin (HCG)

HCG is only present in the body when a woman is pregnant and is the hormone used to detect pregnancy in tests. It is produced by the embryo in the early stages before the placenta takes over. HCG is implicated in the nausea and sickness that affects many women during the early weeks of pregnancy.

Prolactin

Prolactin initiates milk production after the birth and it may have a role in suppressing ovulation while breastfeeding.

Insulin

Insulin, and its corresponding hormone glucagon, are produced in the pancreas and work together to maintain optimal blood glucose levels. Pregnancy places the body in a pre- or mild diabetic state and can lead to gestational diabetes, which affects around 5 per cent of women.

Human Placental Lactogen (HPL)

HPL is produced by the placenta and is similar to human growth hormone in structure and function. It supports the development of the foetus by regulating energy supply and is also involved in milk production.

Endorphins and beta-endorphins

These morphine-like chemicals are released during exercise and promote a sense of well-being as well as decreasing pain perception. Regular exercise in pregnancy helps to increase levels of endorphins and is believed to promote their release during labour which may reduce the perception of pain of childbirth.

Benefits of exercise for the endocrine system

Regular exercise helps to maintain balanced levels of hormones and chemicals in the blood which assist in the smooth functioning of most of the systems of the body, both physiological and psychological, including helping to regulate mood. It can also help to reduce the risk of gestational diabetes and pre- and postnatal depression.

THE CARDIOVASCULAR SYSTEM

The cardiovascular system is responsible for transporting oxygen to the cells of the body and for removing waste products via the bloodstream. The effects of pregnancy on this system are considerable and as the circulation of the mother and baby are interrelated via the placenta, these effects do need to be considered when planning and teaching any form of exercise or physical activity.

Increased resting heart rate

An increase in blood volume results in the heart having to work harder so there is an increase in the heart rate of up to 15 beats per minute over pre-pregnancy levels. There is also an increase in stroke volume, the amount of blood pumped from the heart in one beat, of up to one-third. The result of these two changes means that cardiac output, the amount of blood pumped from the heart in one minute, also increases by up to 50 per cent and the heart muscle, particularly the left ventricle, may increase in size to cope with the extra demand placed on it.

Physiological anaemia

Although blood volume increases, there is not a proportionate increase in the number of red blood cells which means that a type of anaemia, known as physiological anaemia, can occur. This can result in tiredness and fatigue throughout pregnancy and particularly in the first trimester, which may affect motivation to exercise.

Blood pressure in pregnancy

During the first trimester blood volume starts to increase to help with the demands of the growing baby and by the end of the pregnancy it will have increased by between 30 per cent and 50 per cent. However, this takes some time to come about so there may be a short period where there is an inadequate circulating volume of blood to maintain normal blood pressure. This is known as 'vascular underfill' and may lead to dizziness and light-headedness when standing for longer than a few minutes, or when changing from a lying to seated or seated to standing position quickly. This is referred to as postural or orthostatic hypotension and means care should be taken to avoid sudden changes in position or standing still for more than a couple of minutes. Heart rate may also 'race' in order to try and maintain adequate blood pressure in the exercising body.

By the second trimester the body has adapted to the increases in blood volume and cardiac output, and the blood pressure should have normalised. This results in very efficient aerobic function which may lead to improved feelings of fitness and health – often referred to as 'blooming'.

By the third trimester the pressure of the uterus on the vena cava (even when standing), together with reduced vascular tone generally, may lead to oedema (swelling) in the lower legs and ankles, and varicose veins may appear. These typically occur on the lower legs but may also appear in the rectum (piles).

Supine hypotensive syndrome

Supine hypotensive syndrome is an effect on the circulatory system due to the weight of the pregnant uterus. It affects some, not all, pregnant women. If the mother lies on her back (supine) the weight of the uterus and baby can press down on the major blood vessels into and out of the heart (vena cava and aorta). This can inhibit blood flow and make women feel dizzy and nauseous. It is quickly and easily relieved by laying the woman on her side (preferably the LEFT side as the vena cavae are on the right side of the body); however, current guidelines recommend no supine exercise after about 16–20 weeks (ACOG, 2009; RCOG, 2006).

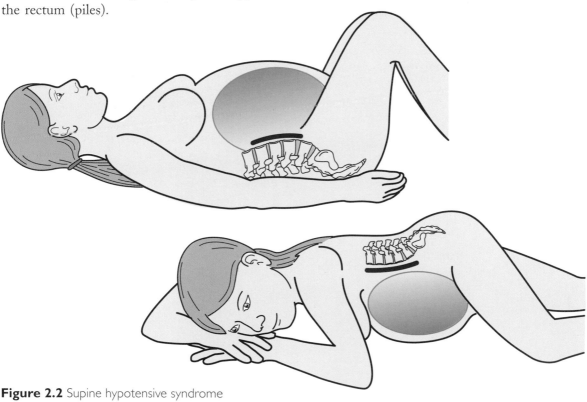

Figure 2.2 Supine hypotensive syndrome

Benefits of exercise on the cardiovascular system

Exercise can help to enhance the already increased stroke volume and cardiac output and improves oxygen transportation to the foetus. It can help to improve or maintain maternal fitness and stamina during pregnancy. A further benefit is that activity, particularly water-based exercise, promotes more efficient venous return which may help to prevent or temporarily alleviate oedema (swelling) and varicose veins in the legs and ankles.

THE RESPIRATORY SYSTEM

The cardiovascular and respiratory systems are linked and any pregnancy-related changes to one system will affect the other. During pregnancy, progesterone makes the respiratory centre in the brain more sensitive to carbon dioxide which, in turn, causes the breathing rate to increase in order to eliminate it. The increased metabolic rate caused by pregnancy requires increased oxygen levels which also affects breathing rate so women may appear to be breathing much faster than in the non-pregnant state. However, although the breathing rate is faster and may appear less efficient, the tidal volume, the amount of air inhaled and exhaled in a single breath, actually increases by up to 40 per cent. This promotes a better uptake and utilisation of oxygen and dissipation of carbon dioxide, making the respiratory system more efficient. The vasodilatory effects of progesterone also affect the smooth muscle tissue in the airways and many women find that pre-existing asthma reduces during pregnancy. Others find their asthma may stay the same or even worsen.

The combined effects of these changes mean that although the respiratory system is more efficient, it can produce an uncomfortable sensation of shortness of breath, even at low levels of activity or exercise. In the second and third trimesters the

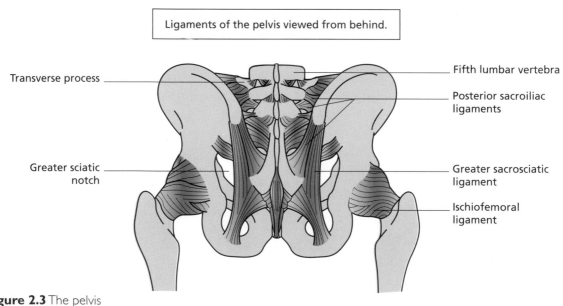

Ligaments of the pelvis viewed from behind.

Transverse process

Greater sciatic notch

Fifth lumbar vertebra

Posterior sacroiliac ligaments

Greater sacrosciatic ligament

Ischiofemoral ligament

Figure 2.3 The pelvis

growing uterus places pressure on the diaphragm and lungs, reducing space for expansion, so shortness of breath may occur at previously manageable intensities of activity.

Benefits of exercise on the respiratory system

Regular exercise in pregnancy helps to maintain aerobic fitness and function and improves the uptake and use of oxygen by both mother-to-be and foetus. A study by Kansas City University of Medicine and Biosciences found that the respiratory system, breathing movement and nervous system of babies whose mothers exercised during pregnancy was better developed and more mature and suggests that the risk of cot death is reduced (May, L. M 2008).

THE MUSCULOSKELETAL SYSTEM

During pregnancy, the musculoskeletal system is affected by the hormone relaxin which relaxes connective tissue. Although the main aim of this hormone is to relax the pelvis to facilitate childbirth, relaxin affects all joints in the body so care needs to be taken to avoid overstretching or over-stressing joints.

The pelvis

During pregnancy the pelvis may become destabilised as the sacroiliac and pubic joints loosen to prepare for childbirth. This starts in the first trimester although the effects are not usually felt until further into pregnancy, often in the later weeks of the second trimester and in the third trimester. However, if the pelvis was affected during previous pregnancies this may occur earlier. As relaxin starts to affect the joints of the pelvis discomfort may be experienced during physical

The pelvis – key points

The pelvis has a number of key functions including transmitting the weight of the upper body to the legs and protecting the pelvic organs, including the uterus. The brim of the female pelvis is rounder and wider than that of males to accommodate the growing foetus in pregnancy.

The pelvis is made up of three bones; two hip bones, the sacrum and the coccyx. The hip (or innominate) bones are each formed from three bones:

- The ilium
- The ischium
- The pubis

There are two key pelvic joints, the sacroiliac joint formed by the junction of the sacrum and ilium at the back, and the pubic symphysis at the front. The sacroiliac joints are covered with cartilage and secured with ligaments which stabilise the joint, (figure 2.3) and the pubic symphysis is connected by a pad of cartilage.

The joints of the pelvis allow a small amount of multi-directional movement.

activity or exercise, particularly on impact or when in wide legged positions.

As the pregnancy progresses and the foetus grows within the abdominal cavity, the pelvis may move into an anterior tilt. The combination of this with the lengthened abdominal muscles and an increased lordotic curve may lead to back pain. This in turn can cause shortening of the hip flexors and lengthening and tightening of the hamstrings. By the third trimester the gap at the pubic symphysis may have increased from 3–4 mm/0.1–0.15 inches to 9 mm/0.35 inches which further destabilises the pelvis and can lead to pelvic girdle pain (PGP) which can occur during activity or even when sedentary. A gap of more than 10 mm/0.4 inches and up to 35 mm/1.4 inches may indicate diastasis symphysis pubis which needs proper investigation, diagnosis and treatment advice from a health care professional before resuming activity.

Benefits of exercise for the pelvis

Regular exercise with an emphasis on pelvic alignment will help to maintain correct posture and keep the ligaments and muscles that support the pelvis strong. This will help prevent or alleviate any aches or pains and may delay or avert pelvic girdle pain. Additionally the muscles that support the spine will be stronger and fitter and promote better posture throughout pregnancy.

The spine

The spine has many joints, all of which may be affected by relaxin as well as by the growing weight of the uterus and breasts. It is never too early to start to focus on correct spinal alignment and posture in pregnancy as the stronger the supporting muscles, the less of an impact there will be on the spine leading to reduced aches and pains.

During the first trimester the main effect will be due to the increasing weight and size of the breasts and if posture was poor previously, there may be an increased kyphotic curve of the thoracic spine. This is likely to develop as the pregnancy progresses and the head and chin may start to protrude forward, the pectoral muscles shorten, trapezius and rear deltoid muscles lengthen, leading to more rounded shoulders.

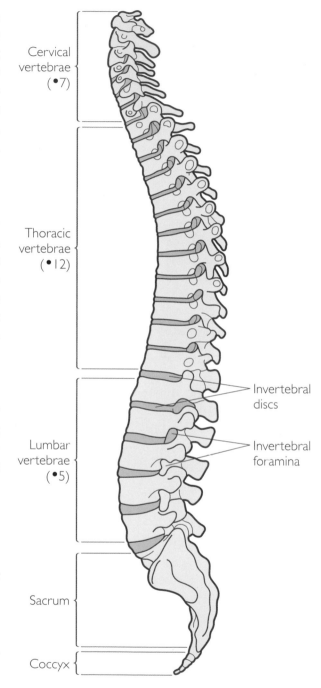

Cervical vertebrae (•7)

Thoracic vertebrae (•12)

Lumbar vertebrae (•5)

Sacrum

Coccyx

Invertebral discs

Invertebral foramina

Figure 2.4 The spine

The spine – key points

The spine has 33 vertebrae which form five sections. There are seven vertebrae in the cervical spine, 12 in the thoracic spine and five in the lumbar spine (figure 2.4).

These three sections have intervertebral discs between each vertebra which maintain alignment and protect from impact.

The base of the spine forms part of the pelvis and is made up of the five fused vertebrae of the sacrum and the four fused vertebrae of the coccyx.

There are four curves in the spine, inward (lordotic) curves in the cervical and lumbar regions and outward (kyphotic) curves in the thoracic and sacral/coccygeal sections. These curves provide shape and shock absorption.

As the foetus grows and the uterus expands out of the pelvis, the weight and change in centre of gravity may cause the lordotic curve in the lumbar spine to increase. The general increase in weight during pregnancy will also place stress on the intervertebral joints and discs, potentially leading to backache, which can range from mild to severe.

The effects of relaxin are at a peak in the third trimester which coincides with the greatest weight and size of the abdomen and breasts. If posture is already compromised, chances are it will get worse now and increase the likelihood of discomfort in the back. Even if good posture has been maintained through most of the pregnancy, it is likely to be affected in the last few weeks.

Benefits of exercise for the spine

An emphasis on exercises that promote good posture before and during pregnancy will help to alleviate some of the effects of pregnancy. However, it is likely that even those women with excellent posture may experience some changes to spine alignment, so minimising these by maintaining strength in the supporting muscles would be an appropriate aim for any activity or exercise programme including aqua-natal sessions.

Other joints

As previously stated, relaxin affects all joints and, other than the possible detrimental effects to the spine and pelvis, the main issue is the risk of hypermobility. During pregnancy, women may feel that their flexibility is improving, however this is due to the joints becoming less stable and so movement needs to be carefully controlled as any overextension of the ligaments or tendons may lead to lasting damage. The feet are particularly affected by relaxin as they bear the weight of the growing body and can flatten and widen and may even increase in size. Well-fitting, comfortable shoes are a must for this reason, particularly when performing any activities that involve low to moderate impact. Although impact is minimised when exercising in water, for any woman experiencing discomfort in the feet, aqua shoes (a type of waterproof trainer) are available to improve support and provide additional cushioning.

Carpal tunnel syndrome

The symptoms of carpal tunnel syndrome may increase if oedema is present in the wrists and this may make gripping or pressure on the wrists uncomfortable (figure 2.5).

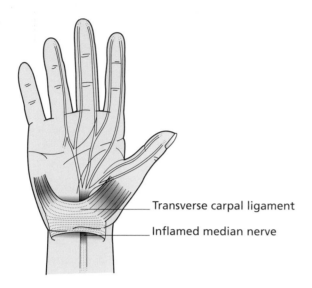

Transverse carpal ligament

Inflamed median nerve

Figure 2.5 The wrist and carpal tunnel syndrome

Benefits of exercise for the joints

Keeping the muscles strong and avoiding over-extension will help to support the joints during pregnancy and prevent or minimise problems afterwards.

The muscles

In general, muscles are affected in pregnancy more due to changes in posture and hypermobility than to specific hormonal effects. However, there are significant changes to the abdominal muscles that need to be considered. The four layers of abdominal muscles together with the muscles at

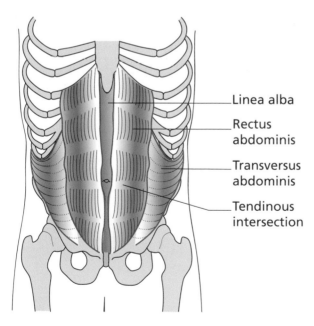

Linea alba

Rectus abdominis

Transversus abdominis

Tendinous intersection

Figure 2.6 The rectus abdominis

Abdominal muscles – key points

In brief, there are four layers of muscles forming a hoop around the torso. From the deepest to the most superficial, these are:

- Transversus abdominis
- Internal obliques
- External obliques
- Rectus abdominis

There are also two fascia, the abdominal fascia (anterior) and lumbodorsal fascia (posterior) which provide tension.

The three deeper layers are covered by, and the rectus abdominis is surrounded by, a sheath of connective tissue called the aponeurosis which joins at the linea alba in the middle of the torso.

As well as these muscles, there are three key muscles at the back which also support the spine:

- Multifidus
- Quadratus lumborum
- Erector spinae

Physiology review: abdominal muscles

The function of abdominal muscles is to:

- provide a protective brace and support for the spine;
- maintain correct pelvic alignment;
- control movements of the torso;
- provide support and protection for the abdominal organs;
- aid expulsive movements e.g. defaecation, coughing;
- support the pregnant uterus;
- assist in expiration

the back form a band around the torso which protects and supports the spine and abdomen and provides movement.

During pregnancy this band supports the growing uterus. However, as the uterus expands and grows out of the pelvis and into the abdominal cavity, these muscles need to adapt to accommodate it. The two sheaths of rectus abdominis lengthen and stretch around the growing abdomen, which weakens them and reduces full support of the uterus. The centre of gravity alters as the uterus grows and protrudes forward, stress on the abdominal and spinal muscles, leading to increased lumbar lordosis and an anterior tilt to the pelvis. The effect of these postural changes is likely to cause stress on the erector spinae muscles, hip flexors and hamstrings and may lead to further deterioration in posture and the increased possibility of back pain. This may be worsened if the anterior tilt of the pelvis and lordotic curve is excessive. By the third trimester the recti bands may have increased in length by

20 centimetres/8 inches, to a possible 50 centimetres/20 inches, with the waist also increasing in size by up to 50 centimetres/20 inches. This may cause the rectus abdominis to separate at the linea alba, leading to a condition called diastasis recti (figure 2.7) which makes the abdominals even less able to provide support to the growing uterus and the spine.

This condition actually occurs in up to two-thirds of women so may be considered a normal feature of pregnancy; however, it does have implications for the muscles postnatally which are discussed later. If the muscles were already in a weakened state, either due to previous pregnancies or obesity, this may occur earlier in pregnancy or be more severe.

Benefits of exercise for muscles

Appropriate exercise will help to prevent excessive damage to the abdominal and back muscles

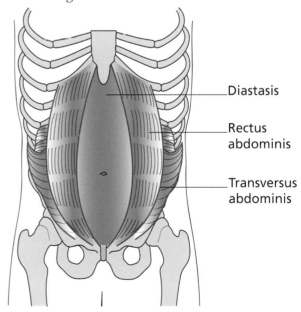

Diastasis

Rectus abdominis

Transversus abdominis

Figure 2.7 Diastasis recti

17

and will help with everyday activity. A whole body approach to muscle strength and endurance in general, with an emphasis on strengthening weaker muscles and stretching tighter ones, will help with everyday activities, promote posture, maintain correct muscle balance and prevent or reduce excessive kyphosis or lordosis and resulting back pain. A strong transversus abdominis will also provide support for the uterus – much like a corset! If the abdominal and back muscles are in good condition then return to the pre-pregnant state after delivery is also likely to be quicker.

The pelvic floor muscles

Although these are part of the muscular system, they deserve to be considered separately as they are often neglected in favour of more visible muscles. Relaxin affects these muscles too which, combined with the weight of the baby pressing down, can lead to incontinence, both bladder and bowel, not only during pregnancy but also for some time afterwards.

The pelvic floor – key points

The pelvic floor (figure 2.8) is a sling of two layers of muscles, deep and superficial, running from the pubic bone to the coccyx and it has two main functions: to support the abdominal contents and to maintain continence.

The pelvic floor muscles contain both fast (approximately 30 per cent) and slow (approximately 70 per cent) twitch fibres. The slow fibres support the abdominal contents and the fast contract in response to changes in intra-abdominal pressure such as coughing, sneezing or laughing.

Benefits of exercise for the pelvic floor muscles

Keeping the pelvic floor muscles in good condition means they will be better able to stretch to facilitate delivery and will be quicker to recover afterwards. Additionally, incontinence is less

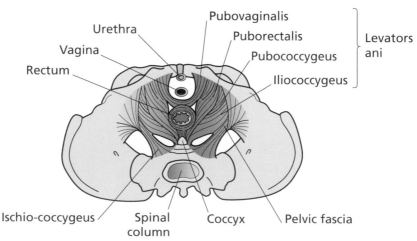

Figure 2.8 The pelvic floor muscles

likely both during and after pregnancy. It is never too early to start pelvic floor exercises – but it is always too early to stop!

THE URINARY SYSTEM

The pelvic floor muscles have a role in the function of the urinary system which is also affected by pregnancy. In the first trimester an increase in urination (or micturition) is common and is caused by the influence of progesterone on the tone of the smooth muscle tissue in the bladder. This results in the bladder attempting to empty even small amounts of urine frequently, but the lack of bladder muscle tone means some urine may be retained which can increase the chance of urinary tract infections. Later in pregnancy, the uterus expands and descends back down into the pelvis ready for delivery. This will compress the bladder and give the mother the sense of having a full bladder and needing to urinate more often.

In addition, exercising in water may make the need to urinate feel more urgent and this may affect the structure of an aqua-natal session. It is estimated that up to two-thirds of women experience incontinence during pregnancy with around 38 per cent still affected three months after delivery. Furthermore, around one-third of women over 40 'put up with' stress incontinence. Research indicates that doing pelvic floor exercises regularly can be effective in reducing stress incontinence and improving control of urge incontinence of both bladder and bowel (Mørkved, 2007).

Benefits of exercise for the urinary system

Performing pelvic floor exercises throughout pregnancy will help with bladder function and health and reduce the risks of both stress incontinence and urinary tract infections. This may also help with recovery after delivery.

THE GASTROINTESTINAL SYSTEM

The combined effects of the hormones of pregnancy can cause nausea, sickness and altered sense of smell and taste. This can range from mild to very severe and many women find that it prevents them being active while others find activity distracts them from these symptoms.

Progesterone's relaxation of the smooth muscle tissue of the body also affects the gastrointestinal system and can make digestion slower. The stomach muscle is less efficient and heartburn and indigestion are common, particularly in the second and third trimesters. Further down the system, the bowel can become more sluggish and

Table 2.3	The two types of incontinence common in pregnancy
Stress incontinence	**Urge incontinence**
• Relaxation or lack of tone in the pelvic floor muscles • Relaxation of smooth muscle tissue of the bladder • Increased abdominal pressure	• Oversensitivity due to bladder infections • Nerve damage • Pressure of foetus • Kicks

stools can become dried out and harder to pass leading to constipation and possible development of rectal haemorrhoids – or piles.

Benefits of exercise on the gastrointestinal system

The beneficial effects of exercise on the gastrointestinal system are well documented and range from improved gastrointestinal transit time (the time taken by food to transit through the system), reduction in constipation and reduction in sensations of nausea and heartburn.

PREGNANCY AND THE METABOLIC SYSTEM

Oestrogen causes a 15–20 per cent increase in the metabolic rate to meet the demands of the growing foetus. This does not, however, mean eating for two since the recommended additional energy intake is only around 300 kilocalories per day – and that only in the second and third trimesters.

Weight gain in pregnancy

During the first trimester the emphasis is on a healthy, balanced diet with a recommended weight gain of only around 1 kg/2.2 lbs, or 8–10 per cent of the total pregnancy weight gain. Any excess energy consumed at this time is likely to be stored as maternal fat. If severe nausea or sickness, or hyperemesis gravidarum (a very severe form of morning sickness) is experienced then weight may actually fall. If this is the case then exercise should not be undertaken and the woman must speak to her health care provider as it is possible to become severely dehydrated.

The greatest weight gain usually occurs in the second trimester, with an average recommended gain of between 6–8 kg/13–17.5 lbs for a woman with a normal pre-pregnancy BMI. This is achieved by continuing with a healthy, balanced diet and adding around 300 kilocalories of good quality food per day. Weight gain in the third trimester is typically slower with a total recommended gain of between 3.5–4 kg/7–9 lbs. Anything less than 1 kg/2.2 lbs per month is very low and should be investigated. Nutritional guidelines are the same as for the second trimester – a healthy balanced diet with an additional 300 kilocalories per day (please note, this is not in addition to the 300 kilocalories in the second trimester!).

Cravings can occur at any time in pregnancy and can range from the relatively normal (ice is a common one) to the strong desire to eat non-food substances such as charcoal or mud! This is known as pica and should resolve after delivery. As long as the cravings are for non-harmful substances then there should be no adverse long-term effects.

The amount of weight gain considered to be healthy varies according to the woman's pre-pregnancy BMI as indicated in Table 2.4.

Table 2.4	Recommended weight gain in pregnancy	
Pre-pregnancy BMI	**Recommended weight gain**	
	Kilograms	**Pounds**
Low < 19.8	12.5–18	28–40
Normal 19.8–26	11.5–16	25–35
Overweight 26–29	7–11.5	15–25
Obese > 29	Minimum 6	Maximum 14

From Medforth et al (2006)

Pregnancy and diabetes

Pregnancy effectively puts the body into a pre-diabetic state as insulin response is slowed to decrease carbohydrate utilisation by the mother and ensure that the foetus has a good supply of carbohydrates. This also helps to preserve fat stores to provide energy in late pregnancy and for lactation after delivery. Women who have type 1 diabetes mellitus or type 2 diabetes mellitus prior to becoming pregnant and who may be receiving additional care, may be more at risk of hypogly-caemia (low blood glucose), particularly in the first trimester (Wahabi, 2012; Visser, 2005; ter Braak et al, 2002).

For non-diabetic women, gestational diabetes mellitus (GDM) can develop if insulin resistance increases too much. This is a form of glucose intolerance occurring in about 1 to 3 per cent of pregnancies and which usually resolves during the extended postnatal period. However, it does indicate an increased risk of developing type 2 diabetes later in life and should be carefully monitored by a midwife during pregnancy.

Benefits of exercise for the metabolic system

Exercise helps to manage weight gain and improves oxygen utilisation. It also helps to improve insulin sensitivity, promoting the use of fat as an energy source, thus maintaining blood glucose levels and reserving carbohydrate stores for the foetus and placenta. This will reduce the risk of hypoglycae-mia and GDM and may improve outcomes of existing GDM (DiNallo & Downs, 2007). Main-tenance of muscle mass by engaging in appropri-ate activity also helps to keep body fat levels at an optimal level and maintains functional ability.

OTHER FACTORS
Thermoregulatory changes

During pregnancy, any increase to maternal core temperature may be harmful to the growing baby. In order to safeguard the baby, a number of changes occur in the mother's body:

* Early in pregnancy, the body's normal 'set point' temperature decreases – similar to turn-ing a thermostat down.

- The effects of progesterone induce vasodilation, resulting in a marked increase in blood flow to the skin. This raises skin temperature on various parts of the body by 2–6 degrees Celsius, meaning that the rate of heat loss directly from the skin is increased.
- Sweating may occur at a lower point than in the non-pregnant state, thus during pregnancy women may start to sweat almost as soon as body temperature starts to rise. Since the skin is already warm, the sweat quickly starts to evaporate and will cool the woman down.
- Heat is also lost to the growing baby and is dissipated through the increased breathing rate.

All of these changes mean that the ability of women to get rid of heat improves so much due to the adaptations of pregnancy that often they have to increase their heat production to stay warm when they are not active (Clapp, 2002).

Breast discomfort

Due to hormone changes breasts may become swollen and very sore. In the later weeks of pregnancy, the breasts start to prepare for feeding the baby and may leak colostrum or 'first milk'. Lots of arm movements or water lapping around the breasts in an aqua-natal session can increase this leakage and make breasts more uncomfortable.

Fear of miscarriage

In the early stages of pregnancy, women may be concerned about the well-being of the baby. They may also be anxious about the months to come and the birth.

There is a higher risk of miscarriage or spontaneous abortion in the first trimester, around weeks 8–12. By this time, all the organ systems of the embryo (now called a foetus) should be in place and the placenta continues to develop. If there are significant defects with the embryo or problems with the placenta, then the pregnancy may naturally terminate at this point. Many women will have very early miscarriages without realising they were ever pregnant. About one in eight pregnancies end in this way. By 12 weeks, if foetal heartbeat is normal or ultrasound is normal, miscarriage risk drops to about 1 per cent.

The nervous system

The main pregnancy related change to the nervous system is slower reaction times, which is further compounded by the growing abdomen and change in centre of gravity. This may make sudden changes of direction or fast-paced movement more challenging. Regular activity will help to maintain motor skills and promote healthy functioning of the nervous system.

Fluid retention (oedema)

Due to hormonal influences, particularly oestrogen, fluid can be retained in the tissues causing oedema, or swelling. This is most obvious in wrists, hands and ankles and can make some

> **IMPORTANT NOTE:**
> Sudden swelling/oedema can be a sign of a very serious complication of pregnancy called pregnancy-induced hypertension (pih) or gestational hypertension. If left untreated, this can lead to a more serious condition called pre-eclampsia. If the woman complains of any sudden swelling she should be referred to a health professional for investigation.

movements uncomfortable, for example wrist flexion in a box press-up position may cause numbness or tingling in the fingers, and standing still for too long can increase swelling in the ankles. Fluid levels in the eyes also change and contact lenses may not fit as well.

Skin

There are a number of ways that skin is affected by pregnancy; the skin over the line of the linea alba darkens and is called the linea negra; the areola and nipples can darken; a blotchy rash, known as chloasma, can appear on the face; skin texture can change, becoming oilier or drier; vasodilation of the vessels to the skin can cause a 'glow'. In addition, stretch marks may appear on the abdomen, thighs or upper body due partly to the stretching of the skin and also to hormones.

Leg cramps

Around one-third of pregnant women experience leg cramps which may be particularly evident at night. Exercise may help prevent these by maintaining muscle tone and circulation.

Thrush

Changes in blood glucose and hormone levels can cause an increase in thrush which can be uncomfortable or cause significant itching. Water-based exercise may not be appropriate as chlorine may increase irritation to the affected areas.

PSYCHOLOGICAL EFFECTS OF PREGNANCY

Pregnancy can have a major impact on emotions; partly due to the disruption of hormones, but also through understandable concerns or worries about the pregnancy, birth and future. This means that mental health conditions may arise during pregnancy and any pre-existing conditions may be exacerbated. It is not easy for a woman to disclose a mental health condition under normal circumstances, so it may be particularly hard during pregnancy when it may be assumed that she 'must be so happy'. For this reason it is worth mentioning briefly some of the mental health conditions more commonly encountered during pregnancy.

Anxiety

While it is perfectly understandable, and possibly 'normal', for a pregnant woman to be anxious about the health of her baby, the actual birth and being able to cope afterwards, it should not be overwhelming or affect everyday life. If this happens it can have a detrimental effect on both the mother and on the pregnancy outcome. If you become concerned about anxiety levels in a client, it is recommended that you suggest she consults her health care provider for advice.

Obsessive Compulsive Disorder (OCD)

OCD is characterised by repetitive behaviours or compulsions, the more common of which are checking, numbering, cleaning and washing. Pre-existing OCD may be exacerbated, and pregnancy-induced OCD may be due to a fear of causing harm to the foetus either through behaviours or through a need for extreme cleanliness.

Depression

There is an understandable focus on postnatal depression as it is a relatively common condition which can adversely affect a woman and her ability to cope with the demands of a new baby. However, some estimates (Evans et al, 2001;

Price 2007) suggest that levels of prenatal depression may be as high as one in three women and possibly even higher. Prenatal depression is hard to diagnose as many women are reluctant to acknowledge that they are feeling low in case they are stigmatised. However, as this may lead to an increased risk of postnatal depression it is important to recognise the symptoms so that you can encourage the woman to discuss any issues with an appropriate health care professional.

The key symptoms of depression include:

- Low mood
- Significantly reduced interest in previously pleasurable activities
- Weight loss
- Insomnia or hypersomnia
- Slowed down or agitated movement patterns
- Fatigue and/or loss of energy
- Feelings of worthlessness or guilt
- Lack of concentration or focus
- Thoughts of death or suicide (NB: there may be no intention to commit suicide)

These symptoms need to have been present for over two weeks, for most of the time and represent a change in normal functioning. It may be difficult to distinguish fatigue and lack of concentration due to depression from some of the 'normal' symptoms of pregnancy (particularly the later stages). However, if there is any concern encourage the woman to discuss her symptoms with her midwife or GP.

Risk factors for prenatal depression include:

- Young age
- Low education levels or achievement
- Low income
- High anxiety
- Body image issues
- Poor self-esteem
- Past history of depression.

Severe and enduring mental health conditions in pregnancy

A woman who develops or has pre-existing conditions such as schizophrenia, bipolar disorder or personality disorder requires specialist mental health care and will be beyond the scope of most instructors. Instructors who want to work with pregnant and postnatal women with a mental health condition are advised to undertake additional training and to work only in conjunction with a qualified mental health professional.

Benefits of exercise for mental health

There is considerable evidence to suggest that activity is valuable in both preventing and alleviating mental health conditions so, provided there are no other contraindications and the condition is considered mild to moderate in effect, exercise is recommended to help boost psychological health during pregnancy.

Pregnancy-associated long-term memory impairment

While the benefits of regular exercise on the brain's function are well evidenced, the effects of exercise and activity on pregnancy-associated long-term memory function are less well known. Studies suggest that water-based exercise, in particular swimming, during pregnancy alleviates the pregnancy-associated decrease in memory function in the longer term (Kim et al, 2012).

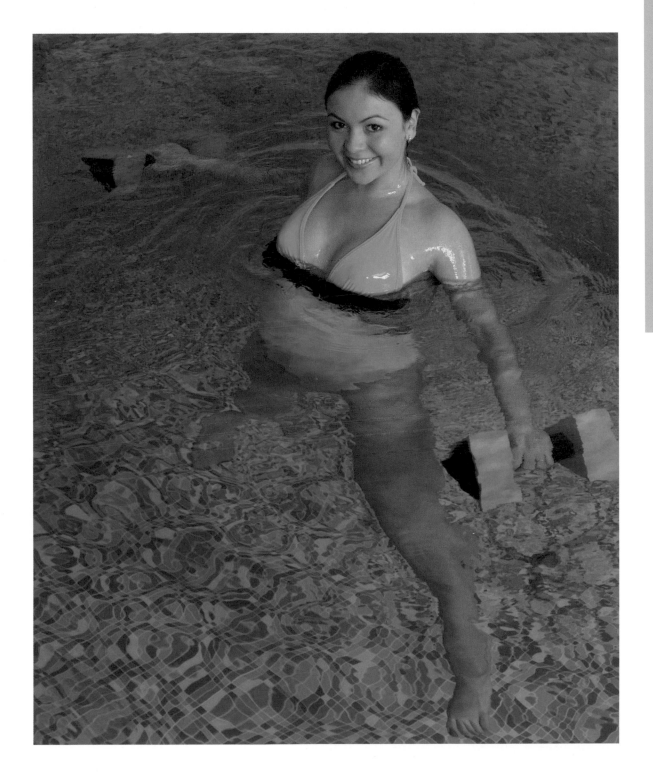

Table 2.5 Summary of the benefits of exercise during pregnancy

Physical benefits

Better pregnancy posture	Including specific exercises, especially for the back and abdominals, reduces the impact of the developing pregnancy on posture. This in turn can help to alleviate or prevent back, neck and shoulder pain.
Better muscle tone	Regular activity will help to maintain or improve muscle endurance and strength during pregnancy, and to support childcare related activities after delivery.
Better circulation	The smooth muscle of blood vessel walls relaxes under the influence of progesterone during pregnancy. By exercising or being active regularly, blood flow can be improved and potentially reduce the formation of varicose veins and development of oedema.
Reduced digestive discomfort	Exercise can help reduce constipation, indigestion and heartburn during pregnancy. A welcome benefit!
Maintenance of bone density	By incorporating weight-bearing activity into a fitness programme, bone density can be maintained throughout the 9 months of pregnancy.
Reduced risk of comorbidities or complications	Exercising during pregnancy can help reduce the risk of gestational diabetes, hypertension or depression.
Better coping ability for delivery	Performing appropriate activity during pregnancy can help to improve fitness in preparation for childbirth. If the client is relatively strong, with good stamina, then she may be able to cope with labour more easily.
Control of weight gain	A certain amount of weight gain is essential in pregnancy. However, excessive weight gain can increase the risk of complications and can exacerbate back and joint pain. Regular exercise can help manage weight gain.
Increased energy and less fatigue	Exercise helps to boost energy levels and relieve feelings of fatigue, which are particularly pronounced in the first and third trimesters.
Less fat on baby	Babies born to exercising women tend to be of similar dimensions (length and head circumference), but have less fat on them than babies born to non-exercisers. This is potentially better for their long-term health as they have a healthier body composition.

Table 2.5	Summary of the benefits of exercise during pregnancy (cont.)
Psychological benefits	
Improved mood	Any physical activity helps to promote better mental health and as prenatal AND postnatal depression rates are increasing, anything that combats this is welcome.
Improved sleep patterns	Regular activity has a beneficial effect on sleep patterns and quality.
Increased self-confidence	Even if a woman is happy to be pregnant and looking forward to the birth of her baby, she might start to feel a bit down about some of the changes that are happening in her body. By helping her maintain good posture and body awareness and allowing her to be in control of her own body again, exercise can improve self-image and confidence.
Social aspect	Exercise in social environments provides the opportunity to meet other pregnant women and share experiences. This may help to reassure women that they are not alone, and what they are going through is natural and normal.
Memory	Reduced or alleviated pregnancy-associated long-term memory function.

THE POSTNATAL PERIOD
LABOUR AND DELIVERY

The majority of women will deliver their babies between 38 and 42 weeks, only 4 per cent are delivered on the estimated due date (EDD) and over 80 per cent appear after the due date, or 'late'. Any baby delivered before 36 weeks is considered premature and after 42 weeks it is likely that delivery will be induced.

Labour

Labour has three stages; stage one is characterised by contractions which help to move the baby down the birth canal and dilate the cervix in preparation for delivery. The second stage is the delivery of the baby, and the third stage is the delivery of the placenta. The type of delivery may impact on when it is suitable for a woman to return to activity.

Normal vaginal delivery

In this type of delivery there is little or no medical intervention, other than pain relief. Recovery rates are typically quick, apart from tenderness or discomfort in the perineum which may remain for several days or weeks.

Traumatic vaginal delivery

If delivery is assisted in some way, either by forceps or a ventouse cup it can result in greater discomfort or pain in the perineal area so recovery may take longer, particularly if an episiotomy or tear occurred during delivery.

Breech presentation

A breech presentation is when the baby is lying with the bottom or feet in the pelvis instead of the head. This occurs in around 3–4 per cent of full term pregnancies. Currently, the majority of babies, and almost all first babies, presenting in the breech position will be delivered by Caesarean section.

Pelvic floor muscles

Any type of vaginal delivery may cause damage to the pelvic floor muscles and this can take time to heal. Starting pelvic floor exercises as soon as possible after delivery will help this process.

Lower segment Caesarean section (LSCS)

A LSCS is when the baby is delivered through an incision in the abdomen and uterus. This can be elective (decided in advance) or as an emergency if there are complications in pregnancy or during labour.

The site of the LSCS incision needs care and any activity should be very gentle to avoid separation or infection.

The new mother and baby may stay in hospital for between a few hours to a few days, depending on complications, while after a home delivery new mothers are advised to rest for a few days to allow the body to recover.

POSTNATAL EFFECTS

The uterus

Within minutes of giving birth the uterus shrinks to the size of a grapefruit and ten to twelve days after birth has returned to the pelvis.

Breastfeeding causes the uterus to contract more forcefully which helps it to shrink back faster; however, these contractions can be uncomfortable, or even painful, and can last for three to four days after starting to breastfeed. The ligaments that support the uterus will return to normal very quickly; however, vigorous exertion or twisting movements in the first few days can result in severe abdominal pain and should be avoided.

The cardiovascular and respiratory systems

The cardiovascular and respiratory systems return to normal soon after birth. Any excess blood volume is converted to fluid and expelled through urination in the first few days after delivery. Breathing will become easier as the lungs and diaphragm now have more room to expand.

The musculoskeletal system

The two bands of the rectus abdominis muscle will start to realign within three or four days of delivery. Provided there are no complications and if appropriate exercises are performed the abdominal muscles can regain tone within a short time.

Relaxin may affect the joints for up to six months, possibly longer if breastfeeding, so care must still be taken to avoid overstretching. The postural changes and the effects of relaxin may have led to considerable backache which may be exacerbated if an epidural was used during delivery. The joints of the spine are still affected by relaxin so the weight of breasts and positions used when breastfeeding may increase the possibility of continued discomfort in the back.

There may be residual pelvic girdle pain, or this may appear now, and could be felt anywhere around the hips, buttocks, thighs, lower back, pubic area or groin. If this is moderate to severe it should be checked by an appropriate health care professional before activity is recommenced.

The pelvic floor muscles are likely to have been weakened or damaged during pregnancy or birth and this can lead to stress incontinence. Over 67 per cent of women report continued stress incontinence three months after delivery. Pelvic floor exercises should be resumed as soon as possible after delivery to help prevent or alleviate this.

The vagina regains its pre-birth tone naturally, but pelvic floor exercises will help speed this up. If stitches were necessary they can take up to six weeks to dissolve and may feel uncomfortable during this time. This discomfort plus any bruising to the coccyx during delivery may make sitting positions uncomfortable.

The nervous and endocrine systems

The hormones of pregnancy return to normal levels soon after delivery and breastfeeding will speed this process up.

It is normal for new mothers to feel exhausted or overwhelmed for a few days, psychologically as well as physically due to the huge physical and emotional demands of pregnancy and childbirth. Around half of new mothers will experience a low period known as 'baby blues' which tends to occur around the third or fourth day after delivery, often when the milk comes in. This can cause weepiness, depression and feelings of being overwhelmed, but this is a relatively normal emotional experience which should pass within a few days. It is also common for new mothers to feel physically tired, anxious and lethargic, but find it hard to sleep.

The gastrointestinal system

With the fall in progesterone levels and the space created by the birth, heartburn and indigestion are reduced. Constipation will also lessen; however, many women are fearful of pain during bowel movements so may 'hang on' which might increase constipation. If haemorrhoids have occurred during pregnancy or delivery they may be very uncomfortable, especially if constipation is present.

The metabolic system

A breastfeeding mother will require an extra 400–600 kilocalories per day, provided from healthy foods, plus an increase in fluid intake to support the production of milk and prevent dehydration. The increased fat utilisation breastfeeding requires helps with the loss of pregnancy weight (remember maternal fat should only be about 3 kg/ 7 lbs anyway) without the need to restrict calories, and moderate exercise will boost this. However, the recommended weight loss guidelines of 0.5–0.75 kg/1–1.5 lbs a week still apply. If the new mother is concerned about not losing weight, keep her focused on health benefits until breastfeeding ceases.

(Note: Although most women find breastfeeding helps with weight loss, it is not the case for all. Keep the focus on healthy eating and health related exercise rather than weight loss until breastfeeding ceases.)

Encourage the wearing of a well fitting bra underneath sports or swim gear to improve support. Tops or bras that compress the breasts should be avoided as they can cause discomfort or increase the risk of infections such as mastitis. Advise feeding or expressing milk prior to exercise in order to reduce the weight and size of breasts while exercising.

The urinary system

The frequency and quantity of urination significantly increases in the first few days after delivery as the body gets rid of the extra blood volume.

OTHER CHANGES
Lochia

There will be several days or weeks of blood loss (lochia) from the site of placental attachment, which is normal. Breastfeeding helps to speed up the healing of the site and reduce the length of the lochia. Women may want to return to gentle aqua exercise or swimming after delivery, but this is not advisable until the lochia has fully ceased as tampons are not suitable during this time.

Periods

Menstrual periods resume between three and eight weeks after birth, or after five or more months if fully breastfeeding. (Note: As ovulation takes place BEFORE the first period occurs women may not be aware that they are pregnant again in the first few weeks after the birth. You need to screen for this as up to 5 per cent of women find out they are pregnant again at their six-week postnatal check.)

COMPLICATIONS OF THE IMMEDIATE POSTNATAL PERIOD
Mastitis

This inflammation of the breast tissue causes the breasts to become red, lumpy and very painful. Mastitis is a potentially serious condition which causes fever and illness. Exercise would not be appropriate or advisable if mastitis is present and women are recommended to seek medical advice as soon as possible.

Carpal tunnel syndrome

Carpal tunnel syndrome (CTS) is caused by compression of the median nerve in the wrist due to fluid retention. Common after pregnancy, it appears to be more severe in breastfeeding women although there is no specific cause. Keeping the wrist elevated and correctly aligned and doing regular wrist and finger mobility exercises will help alleviate symptoms. Carpal tunnel syndrome usually resolves after breastfeeding ceases.

Diastasis recti

The recti sheaths separate during late pregnancy which may have been exacerbated by a large abdomen or excessive weight gain. As the muscles will provide little support until they have realigned correctly, returning to 'sit up' styles of exercise before the gap has reduced to around 3 cm/1.5 in can worsen this and may cause increased pressure on the vertebrae and intervertebral discs leading to backache (see Figure 2.9 for the 'rec check' procedure which tests for abdominal separation).

Infection

The site of stitches of a lower segment Caesarean section incision may become infected, which will prohibit activity until fully healed as exercise during this time may cause the incision site to become misaligned.

RECOMMENDATION FOR ACTIVITY IN THE IMMEDIATE POSTNATAL PERIOD – 0–6 WEEKS

Exercise during the immediate postnatal period should be gentle and gradual and the following activities are recommended:

1. **Testing for abdominal separation – the 'rec check'**

   This will check the degree of separation in the recti sheaths and gauge readiness for returning to abdominal curl-ups. The method for this check is described in detail on p.33.

2. **Transverse pull ins/abdominal hollowing**

   These can be done in a seated, standing, prone or supine lying position and instructions are described in the postnatal exercise section of this book (see page 108).

3. **Pelvic floor exercises**

   The pelvic floor exercises started in early pregnancy should be resumed as soon as possible after delivery to help speed the healing process. Start with ten slow and ten fast contractions three times during the day, building up to five sets a day. As the muscles become stronger, lengthen the 'hold' to ten seconds.

4. **Pelvic tilt**

   A simple pelvic tilt performed in a supine lying position can help to return the abdominal muscles to normal. Instructions for this exercise are described in more detail in the exercise section of this book (see page 88).

5. **Back care and posture emphasis**

   The focus should be on maintaining correct postural alignment in all positions, particularly while breastfeeding or pushing a buggy, to help prevent back problems. In addition, the lifting, holding, carrying and twisting techniques taught during pregnancy should be continued.

6. **Walking**

   Gentle walking every day is the ideal activity for a new mother, progressing gradually to a brisk pace while pushing the baby in a pram or pushchair. Avoid pushing a heavy buggy up steep hills in the immediate postnatal period to reduce the risk of vaginal or uterine prolapse.

EXERCISE IMPLICATIONS FOR THE EXTENDED POSTNATAL PERIOD

It is recommended that structured exercise is not restarted until after the six-week check has taken place and the 'all-clear' is given. Following this, a return to pre-pregnancy exercise can be gradually started. However, there are a number of contraindications to activity in the extended postnatal period (post-six weeks) that need to be considered before any activity is started. These are described below.

Once the postnatal check has been carried out, usually about six weeks after delivery for a normal birth and between six and ten weeks for a traumatic or lower segment Caesarean section birth and, providing no problems have been identified, a gradual return to exercise is fine. However, not all areas carry out a postnatal check so you will need to re-screen very carefully if this is the case.

Remember that the client will probably have lost some aerobic fitness or muscular strength and endurance so a gradual return to any pre-pregnancy exercise programme is necessary.

COMPLICATIONS OF THE EXTENDED POSTNATAL PERIOD

There are a number of complications of the postnatal period that may affect participation in exercise generally and water-based exercise in particular.

Diastasis recti – issues and advice

The sheaths of rectus abdominis start to realign within three to four days of delivery if there are no complications. If pre-pregnancy tone was good, abdominal muscles can regain their fitness through appropriate exercise within a relatively short time. It is important to carry out the rec check already mentioned to check for diastasis recti and to identify which exercises are appropriate. This is described in detail in figure 2.9. If the rec check shows that the recti sheaths have realigned sufficiently, women can start to introduce some modified curl-ups into their exercise programme, provided they start gradually and progress slowly. If the sheaths have not realigned properly, abdominal exercises that involve forward flexion may exacerbate diastasis recti or delay its return to normal, so the exercises recommended for the immediate postnatal period should be continued. Perform the rec check at regular intervals and when the sheaths have come together standard abdominal exercises such as curl-ups and modified plank can be added to the programme.

Lower segment Caesarean section (LSCS) issues and advice

During a standard LSCS delivery an incision of about 10 cm is made along the 'bikini' line.

Normally this incision will not cut through any of the abdominal muscles; it usually involves an incision through the single layer of the aponeurosis (connective tissue) in that area. The recti sheaths can then be drawn apart manually, creating space for the baby to be delivered. After delivery, the muscles are realigned and should recover in the same way as they would after a vaginal delivery; the damage to the abdominal muscles is actually less severe than many people assume. Although there may be numbness and tingling felt around the incision, this is part of the normal healing process and the underlying layers of muscle should not be affected.

Contracting the transversus abdominis (TVA) may be painful or uncomfortable while the incision is healing and this may prevent effective engagement of this muscle. However, if there is minimal pain during TVA contraction, these exercises should be started as soon as practical after delivery and certainly by the extended postnatal period. These contractions will help to increase blood flow to the area and facilitate the healing process.

Avoid extreme or rapid twisting and side-bending activities on land or in the pool, for

Testing for abdominal separation

Lie flat on the floor with the knees bent and feet about hip-width apart. Place two fingers sideways with the palm towards the face just below (or above) the navel and press gently into the abdomen.

Inhale then exhale and curl the head and shoulders off the floor. As you hold ths position feel for the two recti bands closing around the fingers. If you feel tension from the bands it is safe to start doing some gentle spinal flexion exercises (curl ups).

If there is no pressure on the fingers or you need to use more than two fingers, the bands are not sufficiently realigned to continue with the pull ins and pelvic tilts until they are realigned. Do this check weekly until they are realigned.

example twisting jumps or side bends with aqua dumbbells. These activities may further stretch muscles that are already weakened and lengthened. Keep the focus on posture throughout the session and include contraction work for the transverse abdominals.

Trapped air within the abdominal cavity as a result of a LSCS may add to post-operative discomfort. This can be helped by gentle pelvic tilts in a supine position on land, but this is quite an advanced exercise in the pool so may need to be adapted for those not used to it. Use a noodle under the shoulders (and possibly the hips if the woman has trouble floating) to perform this more comfortably.

Musculoskeletal issues and advice

The joints will be affected by relaxin for several months following delivery. The pelvis and spine in particular may ache or be painful and the coccyx may have been bruised during labour so sitting or pressure on this area for any length of time may be uncomfortable.

Buoyancy reduces body weight in the water, so stress on the back, pelvis and other weight-bearing joints is reduced. This can help reduce the risks of joint instability. Impact through joints is lessened, again reducing the risks to lax joints (Kihlstrand et al, 1999; Smith & Michel, 2006; Katz, 1996).

Be careful with any extreme range of movement and avoid rocking the hips or twisting the pelvis from side to side; for example, keep side steps small, leg lifts and knee lifts should stay below hip height and any twisting of the hips should be avoided. Avoid prolonged standing on one leg, especially with the pelvis out of alignment, tilted or twisted, and avoid exercises that place the legs in a wide position such as plies or wide squats. Movements that involve the adductors/abductors, for example 'scissor legs', may cause or increase pain in the symphysis pubis, so advise small ranges of movement initially or choose a different exercise. Stretches around the hip area will need to be performed with care too, to ensure that tendons and ligaments are not being stretched beyond a safe range.

Continue to take care with range of movement for all activities. Although the buoyancy and resistance of the water help to support limbs, women may still be able to lock out knees and elbows more easily and turn ankles due to joint laxity. Observe participants carefully to make sure they are not hyperextending any joints.

Exercises that work muscles in conjunction with opposing or stabilising muscles (sometimes referred to as the 'oblique sling') will help to re-align and stabilise the pelvis and should be encouraged as the mother progresses with her fitness. For the back, this involves working latissimus dorsi and the opposing gluteus maximus together – for example, 'superman' style exercises on land, 'cross country ski' (opposite arm and leg) in the pool. For the front, the internal obliques, transversus abdominis and opposing adductors work together in exercises such as opposite arm and leg slide on land, and leg kick to the front with opposite arm touch in the pool. It is recommended that you work with the support of a physiotherapist who specialises in women's health before attempting to prescribe exercise for clients who have symphysis pubis misalignment or any pelvic girdle pain.

Psychological changes

Most new mothers feel exhausted for a few days or much longer, psychologically as well as physically, and the huge physical and emotional demands of pregnancy and childbirth may be overwhelming.

Around half of new mothers experience 'baby blues' which tends to occur when the milk comes in around the third or fourth day after delivery. Women may also feel tired, anxious and lethargic and find it hard to sleep. The combination of these factors can cause weepiness, depression and a sense of being overwhelmed. However, this is a normal emotional experience and should pass within a few days. If it continues for longer than expected it may be helpful to discuss symptoms with a health care professional to make sure any more significant problems are identified and managed.

Postnatal depression (PND) is a serious condition and while it is estimated that anywhere between 5 and 20 per cent of women experience significant PND, this may be the tip of the iceberg. Symptoms are similar to those for depression; however, these often go undetected as the new mother may try to hide it from family and friends out of guilt or shame. It can be very hard when everyone is telling you how happy you must be, to admit that, actually, things are not good or that you are not coping. It can be easy to withdraw from others at a time when you need them most. PND most commonly occurs around three to six months after delivery although it can occur any time in the first two years. It is recommended that medical advice is sought as soon as possible to promote full recovery. If you believe a client is experiencing PND encourage her to seek appropriate help. It may be useful to keep a stock of leaflets covering PND for your participants to take away.

Any form of exercise, including aqua, can have a positive impact on mental health, and the social stimulus of being around other new mothers, who may be experiencing similar emotions, can help promote mental health.

Incontinence

The weight of the uterus and baby combined with the effects of progesterone may have had a negative effect on the pelvic floor muscles and may result in incontinence. The hydrostatic pressure of the water may also encourage urination. Advise participants to empty their bladders before the class and provide regular opportunities during the session. While it may not be practical to keep getting in and out of the pool, it is important that they do! Pelvic floor exercises should be done regularly, in the class and at home to alleviate any symptoms of incontinence (Bo & Finckenhagen, 2003).

Carpal tunnel syndrome

Carpal tunnel syndrome (CTS) is caused by compression of the median nerve in the wrist due to fluid retention. It is common after pregnancy and appears to be more severe in breastfeeding women although it is not known why. Keeping the wrist elevated and correctly aligned will help alleviate symptoms, as will wrist and finger mobility exercises. Carpal tunnel syndrome usually resolves after breastfeeding ceases.

There are both benefits and cautions for water-based exercise (Katz, 2003; Katz, 1996; Kent et al, 1999). The hydrostatic pressure of water can temporarily relieve swelling (oedema), making wrists, hands and ankles more comfortable and improving the symptoms of carpal tunnel syndrome. However, using handheld equipment in the session or performing exercises that put weight through the wrists may aggravate the condition. Avoid excessive pressure on the wrists and prolonged gripping of equipment; instead, alternate exercises requiring handheld equipment with an activity requiring no gripping of equipment.

The breasts

Women who are breastfeeding in the postnatal period will probably have larger and more tender, possibly even painful, breasts. Recommend that a well-fitting sports bra with separate 'formed' cups, or nursing bra, is worn under the swimsuit, making sure that neither item compresses the breasts as this can lead to infections. Key implications for exercise are choice of positions and intensity levels. Lying on the front (or back) may be very uncomfortable and vigorous arm movements can cause milk to leak from the breasts. The depth of water should be considered as it needs to be above or below the breast to avoid discomfort; water lapping over the breast can also cause leakage so it is recommended that breastfeeding mothers exercise after feeding to avoid this.

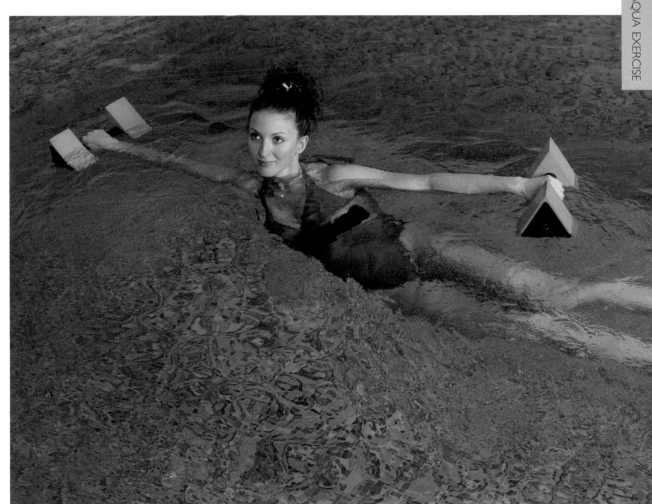

PROPERTIES
OF WATER

3

The aim of this chapter is to review the underpinning knowledge of the properties of water before discussing these in relation to pregnant women. Water has a number of attributes that need to be considered when planning any activity or exercise session in the water. If used appropriately, these properties can make water-based exercise invigorating, safe and fun for a wide range of participants and especially pregnant women.

BUOYANCY

This is the 'up-lift' experienced in water that gives the impression that the body is lighter in water than in air. In water, gravity initially will pull the body down. Then, as the body starts to sink, the pressure of water underneath it increases and creates an up-thrust out of the water. The effects of buoyancy include:

- Body feels lighter (up to 90 per cent reduction in body weight at neck depth, 50 per cent reduction at waist depth, 20–30 per cent reduction at calf/knee depth, when static)
- Decreased impact on joints
- Less stress on joints
- Support for limbs
- Decreased balance/stability

- Increased need for abdominal control to stabilise the body
- Improved range of movement
- May help to decrease heart rate by about 15–20 beats per minute in conjunction with hydrostatic pressure of the water. For this reason, the use of heart rate monitoring may not be such a reliable way of measuring intensity in water as it is on dry land.

Thus, buoyancy is a property that can be used to assist, support or even resist movement in water.

Most aqua-natal classes take place with women submerged in water anywhere between xiphisternum (the lowest end of the sternum, situated just below the centre of the breasts) and shoulders, with feet on the bottom of the pool. Therefore, although not completely weightless, they will feel the benefit of reduced impact through their lower limbs, but may experience less stability at times, as they perform activities in the water.

BUOYANCY, BODY TYPE AND PREGNANCY

The lifting force of buoyancy affects different people in different ways, especially related to the amount and distribution of body fat and muscle.

It is therefore important to visually assess your participants, since body type will affect how water-based activities and exercises are performed and perceived. For example, endomorphs, with a higher percentage of body fat, may be more buoyant and potentially more unstable than mesomorphs who are more muscular, thus travelling through the water may require more effort, whilst floating activities may feel more comfortable. Ectomorphs, being taller and leaner, may find travelling through water easier than trying to stay afloat.

The pregnant uterus, which is largely made up of water, tends to make floating easier. So even those women who had a previous tendency to sink might find this changes during pregnancy.

HYDROSTATIC PRESSURE

This is the pressure exerted by the water on the body. It is a bit like a gentle pressure bandage around the body and has an effect on a number of body systems:

1. If a person is standing vertically in water at about 1.22 metres/4 feet deep, the hydrostatic pressure at the feet is greater than diastolic blood pressure which means venous return to the heart is boosted, and this can be helpful in temporarily reducing peripheral swelling (oedema) and fluid retention in the ankles and feet (Becker, 2011). In non-pregnant women, there can be as much as 700 ml of fluid in the tissues that is redistributed back into the veins within a few seconds of immersion up to neck depth which helps reduce swelling (Greenleaf, 1984).

2. The external hydrostatic pressure displaces blood away from the limbs and increases central blood volume and the amount of blood returning to the heart. This increases the force of contraction of the heart and stroke volume. This increase in stroke volume may be up to 35 per cent if the person is in water up to neck level (Weston et al, 1987). This contributes to the heart rate and blood pressure of individuals exercising in water, including pregnant women, being lower than during land-based exercises.

3. The redistribution of tissue fluid back into the circulatory system increases blood volume and this, together with increased central circulation, means that blood flow to the kidneys is maintained and there is a temporary diuretic (leading to increased urine output) effect. This may necessitate women leaving the pool during the session for a toilet break. Consider structuring the workout to include times when they can do this without interrupting the overall 'flow' of their session.

4. The pressure of water around the chest wall has the overall effect of increasing the work of the respiratory muscles (primarily the inspiratory muscles) by about 60 per cent if submerged at neck depth (Becker, 2011).

This may help to improve respiratory function and could be particularly beneficial for pregnant women hoping to use the birthing pool. Be aware though, that for some individuals who may already have a respiratory condition the hydrostatic pressure on the thorax may limit chest expansion and make breathing more difficult. In addition, any feeling of tightness around the chest may increase anxiety in some participants.

RESISTANCE

Water can provide around 12 to 15 times more resistance than air. This is a constant resistance against which the body needs to work when moving in water. Since this resistance increases as water depth increases, deep water workouts tend to be more challenging than shallow water exercise. This resistance also has significant effects on how muscles work in water (see Muscle Actions and Use of Equipment in Water, page 41). Resistance is also increased by turbulence which means that a large class of people, particularly pregnant women, may create a considerable amount of turbulence and therefore experience more resistance to their movements. This resistance is usually overcome by using propulsion to push the body through the water by exerting force from the arms, legs and torso.

The main types of resistance that need to be considered when planning and teaching a session in the pool are frontal resistance and eddy drag.

Frontal resistance

Because water is denser than air there is increased resistance when moving in any direction. This is called frontal resistance, and it has several effects:

- Activities in water are about three times harder than on land due to the added resistance of water.
- Speed of movement decreases.
- Larger surface area (size of person/use of equipment) and increased speed can provide greater intensity.
- Without equipment, most movements will use both muscles equally within a pair – dual concentric moves. Concentric moves are where the muscle is shortening to overcome resist-

ance. For example, on land a biceps curl will be concentric as the muscle contracts to flex the elbow and lift the forearm, but eccentric as the muscle lengthens and the elbow extends back to a straight arm. However, in water, the movement will be a concentric biceps contraction on the way up and a concentric triceps contraction on the way down.

- In order to create directional movement, participants will have to overcome this water resistance by exerting force from the body (arms, legs and torso) as propulsion.

Hand positions, resistance and propulsion: Use of arms and hands to create propulsion is crucial in facilitating effective movement in water. There are a number of different hand positions that can be adopted that will aid propulsion and can change the intensity of the activity:

1. Cupped hands with fingers closed – water is scooped, pushed or pulled. Very effective for propulsion and sculling, can feel like harder work for the arms.

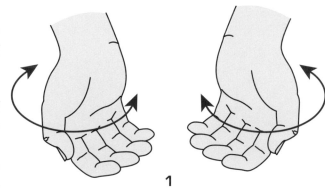

1

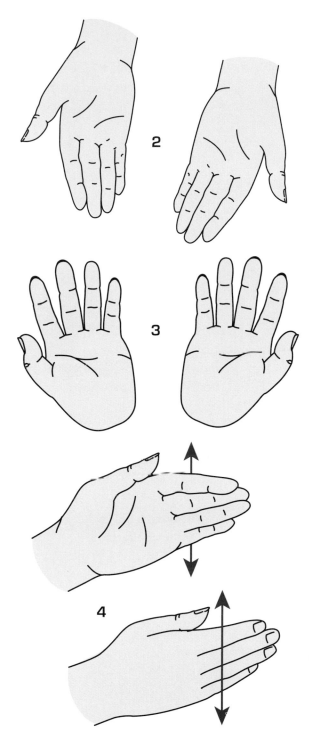

2. Open hands, fingers closed – not so effective for propulsion, increased surface area means increased resistance and potentially harder work for the arms.

3. Open hands, open fingers – not so effective for propulsion, decreased surface area means decreased resistance and potentially less intense work for the arms.

4. Slicing hands (palms open and parallel to direction of arm movement) – not so effective for propulsion, decreased surface area means decreased resistance and potentially less intense work for the arms.

5. Fist (hands clasped in a loose fist) – slight increase in surface area, increases effort.

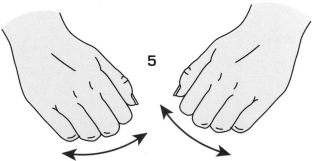

Eddy and drag force

Eddy is the turbulence that forms around and behind the body when moving. In addition, as water flows behind the body, it creates a drag force on the body which tends to pull a person or object backwards (see figure 3.1). As the person or object moves more quickly, eddy and drag force are increased, creating more resistance to movement and changes in direction. This additional resistance has some specific effects; it:

- decreases the ability to change direction quickly;

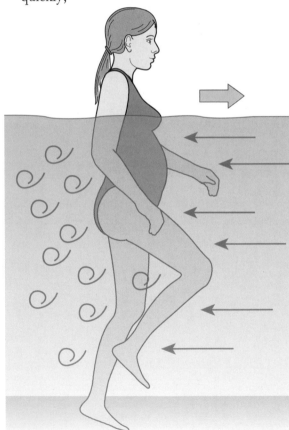

- can help with balance/stability, for example sculling (circling hands or moving hands in a 'figure of eight' to create a mini eddy current).

Thus, for pregnant women who may be experiencing more resistance to movement in water due to frontal resistance, as well as slowing activities down, the addition of transition movements 'on the spot' before changing direction may help to overcome eddy drag. Moreover, if they are feeling a little unbalanced in the water due to buoyancy effects, the use of cupped hands to scull may help them maintain a more steady, stable position.

Other forms of resistance
Viscosity and surface tension

Viscosity of water will resist movement as the molecules of water 'stick' to each other and the person or the object moving through it. As with eddy and drag force, viscosity increases as the person or object moves more quickly. Temperature also affects viscosity and greater viscous resistance will be experienced in a cooler pool.

Surface tension is a force created at the interface between air and water, whereby the surface of the water acts like a skin and can resist movement when a body or limb is moved out of the water into the air or vice versa. This can make it feel harder when moving the arms or body in and out of the water as it takes a bit more effort to get through this 'skin'. This is shown in photographs of swimmers as they come up for air and look like they are in a water bubble.

TEMPERATURE

Water is good at conducting heat away from the body and is much more efficient at doing this than air. This provides a cooling effect on

Figure 3.1 Eddy and drag force

participants, making it unlikely that they will get as hot and sweaty as they might in the gym or aerobics studio. The following are important when instructing an aqua-natal session. It is important to:

- Ensure that participants do not become over fatigued, since they may not realise how hard they are actually working.
- Plan to keep the group moving throughout the session. If static exercises are included, ensure that dynamic activities are included in-between, to warm the group up again.
- Encourage participants to keep moving throughout the session, as remaining still for any length of time will mean they may get cold.
- Make sure that participants continue to drink water frequently during the session.

The ideal temperature for aqua-natal exercise sessions is 29–30 degrees Celsius, with a maximum of 32 degrees Celsius (ACPWH, 2004, 2005). Most leisure centre and health club pools operate between 30 and 31 degrees Celsius. Cooler water may help to decrease heart rate response to exercise, which is another reason why using heart rate monitoring may not be such a reliable way of measuring intensity during water-based exercise as it is on dry land.

DEPTH

All of the above water properties are increased with increasing depth.

The ideal depth for an aqua-natal session is between chest and shoulders, keeping the arms underwater. At the xiphisternum (bottom of the breastbone), the abdominal corset is supported but the upper body may remain cool. As the water reaches the shoulders, the upper body stays warmer and arms can be used effectively under the water, but buoyancy increases and this will challenge stability and balance.

Remember that even if the pool is all one depth, people of different heights will experience different levels of buoyancy and resistance. Shorter individuals will be more deeply submerged and potentially more buoyant. Taller people will experience less buoyancy and resistance but more impact as less of their body is supported by water.

MUSCLE ACTIONS AND USE OF EQUIPMENT IN WATER

Due to the frontal resistance experienced in water, all movements in water without equipment are concentric; there is no eccentric phase. For example, as previously discussed, the biceps will work concentrically in the lifting phase of a biceps curl but the triceps are working concentrically on the lowering phase. This resistance is the same throughout the full range of the movement.

Equipment

There is a variety of equipment that can be used to enhance muscle work in the water. This includes equipment that can increase resistance by increasing the surface area such as mitts and floats. There is also a range of buoyant equipment that requires muscle work to control the movement under the water and may also increase surface area. Types of buoyant equipment include aqua dumbbells, noodles and floats.

If buoyant equipment is used in water, then the opposite muscle group is used to that on dry land. In addition, there will be an eccentric muscle action when the muscle lengthens. Note: This only applies if the equipment is being used in a vertical direction, i.e. up and down, not horizontally.) For example, the biceps arm curl.

This has a number of implications when planning a session:

Table 3.1	Comparing muscle actions		
	ON LAND	**IN WATER** (with no equipment)	**IN WATER** (with buoyant dumbbells)
		Dual concentric move	Opposite muscle used
Upward phase	Biceps concentric	Biceps concentric	Triceps eccentric
Downward phase	Biceps eccentric	Triceps concentric	Triceps concentric

- When exercising without equipment, moves are dual concentric so water-based exercise is a great way of achieving a balanced toning programme for muscles, since flexors and extensors can be worked in the same movement.
- The eccentric phase of contraction tends to be responsible for muscle soreness. If equipment is not used, eccentric contractions are eliminated and therefore soreness post exercise is reduced. It may be necessary to let your participants know this, as some of them may associate sore muscles with an effective workout!
- Particularly when using equipment, stability may be reduced. This will increase the need for fixator (the muscles that hold the rest of the body still) work. In particular, deep abdominal muscles will be required to stabilise the body and maintain balance when standing in water. For pregnant women whose abdominal muscles may already be stretched and weakened, this creates additional work for these muscles. Consider limiting the duration of exercises with equipment so these muscles are not over-fatigued.

- If performing toning work whilst static, it is important to keep the group warm using some dynamic, aerobic moves in between sets/exercises.

Try this practical exercise:

Muscle Actions Exercise
Get yourself in the pool with some equipment and try these exercises.

Table 3.2	Muscle actions exercise					
Exercise	**Upward movement**	**Muscle(s)**	**Action (concentric or eccentric)**	**Downward movement**	**Muscle(s)**	**Action (concentric or eccentric)**
For example, Hamstring curl – no equipment	Flexion	Hamstrings	Concentric	Extension	Quads	Concentric
Lateral raise with aqua dumbbells						
Side leg raise standing upright						
Knee raise with foot on noodle						
Leg kicks						
Upright row with aqua dumbbells						

WHY WATER-BASED EXERCISE?

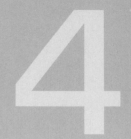

There are a number of benefits of water-based exercise for both the general population and pregnant women. These are summarised below and discussed in more detail on the following pages.

GENERAL BENEFITS OF WATER-BASED EXERCISE

The benefits of aquatic training for the general population typically include improved cardio-vascular fitness, strength, endurance, flexibility and core stability, as well as the social element of working in a group and being able to chat (Lawrence, 2004). Key benefits of water-based exercise include:

- Temperature: water conducts heat more than air, so participants keep cool whilst working hard.
- Buoyancy: the effect of buoyancy when exercising in water provides 'weightlessness' and causes less stress on joints for any participant, particularly those who are overweight or obese. This is also a bonus for heavily pregnant women.
- Provides an effective, low-risk workout with no/minimal impact.
- Water supports movement – it is difficult to fall over in the water! However, be aware that some of the properties of water affect balance.
- Water has a calming effect, providing an unstressed environment.
- Water is a refreshing and exhilarating medium to use.
- Pressure of water aids venous return and helps improve circulation.

GENERAL BENEFITS OF WATER-BASED EXERCISE IN PREGNANCY

Benefits of aquatic training specific to pregnant women include (Smith & Michel, 2006; Parker & Smith, 2003):

- Enhanced physical functioning and mobility
- Reduction in stress in the mother, leading to improved foetal outcome
- Improved body image and health-promoting behaviours.

This last point is borne out by research into weight gain interventions for pregnant obese women. Women expressed positive experiences of a weight gain intervention and had changed their eating and exercise patterns during pregnancy. Almost all had continued with their new patterns after pregnancy. Of these women over

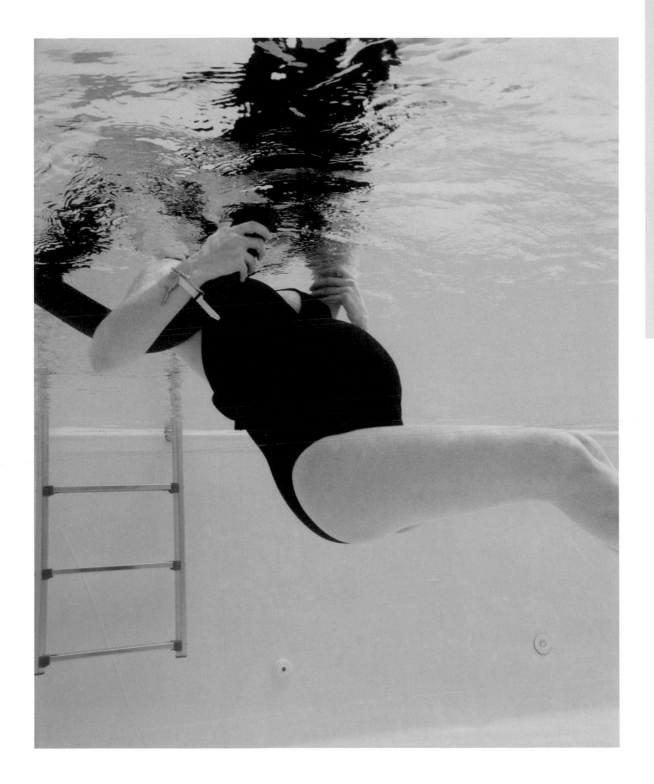

70 per cent took part in aqua aerobic sessions and stated they were most satisfied with this type of exercise and felt that it was a positive social experience (Claesson et al, 2008).

The Women's and Infants' Research Foundation in Australia found that pregnant women participating in swimming training during the second trimester doubled their distance swum and their aerobic fitness increased significantly. Heart rates and blood pressure are lower in water compared to when exercising on land with less effect on foetal heart rate (Katz, 1996). In fact, six out of seven foetuses displayed tachycardia following land-based exercise, with only one in seven following water-based exercise (Katz et al, 1990).

THE PHYSIOLOGICAL BENEFITS OF WATER-BASED EXERCISE IN PREGNANCY

Cardiovascular benefits

Cardiovascular function is enhanced as it allows more efficient uptake and use of oxygen. Venous return is improved which has a beneficial effect on circulation and this may reduce the effects of vascular underfill. Central blood volume and uterine blood flow also increase which preserves blood flow to the baby during the aqua-natal session. Blood pressure and heart rate responses to exercise are reduced.

The potential for supine hypotensive syndrome is reduced by the uplift and lack of gravity in the water. However, abdominal work such as curl-ups on a noodle should be avoided as these could lead to abdominal stretching and may increase the risk or effects of diastasis recti.

The hydrostatic pressure of water can have a temporary beneficial effect on oedema (swelling of tissues due to fluid retention), which is common in later pregnancy. Hydrostatic pressure also has a diuretic (increased urine output) effect after 30–40 minutes in the water which may lead to the need to urinate more frequently. This lasts for up to four hours after the session. However, it is still important to encourage regular hydration during the session.

The respiratory system

As mentioned above, uptake and utilisation of oxygen may be enhanced. The effects of pregnancy on respiratory function are not compounded by immersion and experience of hydrostatic pressure on the chest may be useful if a water birth is planned.

However, if hydrostatic pressure on the chest is uncomfortable or causes anxiety, move the woman to shallower water or to the side of the pool for increased support/confidence.

The musculoskeletal system
The back and spine

Buoyancy reduces body weight resulting in reduced stress on the back, pelvis and other weight-bearing joints. This can help reduce the risks of joint instability and pelvic girdle pain and can also help reduce any aches and pains associated with postural changes; additionally it has been shown to reduce low back pain and absence from work secondary to back pain (Kihlstrand et al, 1999). Evidence suggests that water-based exercise is beneficial to women with chronic pre-existing or pregnancy-related low back pain (Waller and Johan, 2009).

The joints

Impact through joints is reduced during water-based exercise, which reduces the risks to unstable joints. Furthermore, water resistance controls range of movement, and supports and reduces the risk of hyperextending potentially unstable joints.

To avoid any issues with the pelvis, be careful with any extreme range of movement – for example, keep side steps small, keep leg lifts and knee lifts below hip height, offer support at poolside for exercises requiring balance.

Stretches around the hip area will need to be performed with care too, to ensure that tendons and ligaments are not being stretched.

The abdominal muscles

The resistance of the water offers support for the expanding, unstable body with its altered centre of gravity and, combined with hydrostatic pressure and buoyancy, can help to support the abdominal muscles and reduce the risk of diastasis recti. Avoid extreme twisting and side bending activities that may further stretch muscles that are already weakened and lengthened. Focus on posture throughout the session and include education about using the transverse abdominals.

Take care with range of movement for all activities. Although the buoyancy and resistance of the water help to support limbs the woman may still be able to lock out knees and elbows more easily and turn her ankles due to joint laxity, so observe participants carefully to make sure they are not hyperextending any joints. Give frequent verbal reminders too. Encourage good posture throughout the session – engaging deep abdominal muscles around the baby, tucking the pelvis down, lifting the ribcage and keeping the back and neck long.

Carpal tunnel syndrome

Hydrostatic pressure of water can temporarily relieve swelling (oedema), making wrists, hands and ankles more comfortable and improving the symptoms of carpal tunnel syndrome.

Using handheld equipment in the session or performing exercises that put weight through the wrists may aggravate the condition. Try to avoid excessive pressure on the wrists and prolonged gripping of equipment; for example, alternate exercises using handheld equipment with an exercise requiring no equipment.

Thermoregulation

Thermoregulation is reduced when exercising in water as heat is dissipated more easily which reduces the risk of the foetus overheating.

Water temperature of 29–30 degrees Celsius is ideal for prenatal aqua sessions and the surrounding air should be about 1 degree Celsius higher for comfort when participants exit the pool. Cooler water could leave participants feeling chilled; warmer water may lead to vasodilation, hypotension, fainting and fatigue (hospital hydrotherapy pools may be too warm at 36 degrees Celsius or more).

Breast comfort

Water depth is important for breast comfort. If water is under or completely over the bust, it can offer support. If the water level is across the bustline, the pressure of the water lapping around the breasts may become uncomfortable.

A well-fitting supportive bra is essential, even under a swimming costume. It will need to be replaced as the pregnancy progresses and the breasts change size and shape.

Consider keeping arm and upper body activities within a smaller range and shorter duration too.

The digestive system

The massaging effect of water may improve gastrointestinal transit and reduce constipation. However, the pressure of the water may cause an increase in the sensation of feeling full and exercises such as curl-ups on a noodle may increase acid reflux because of compression.

If the woman is feeling nauseous, encourage her to eat a light snack before exercise and rehydrate regularly during exercise to help alleviate symptoms.

Avoid positions that may increase symptoms – for example, forward leaning or curled up.

Table 4.1	Overview of the benefits of water-based exercise in pregnancy	
Pregnancy effect	**Benefits of aquatic training**	**Potential issues and advice**
Vascular underfill	• Reduced effect of vascular underfill • Increased blood volume and uterine blood flow • Reduced exercise blood pressure and heart rate response	• Dehydration – ensure adequate hydration
Supine hypotensive syndrome	• Reduced potential for supine hypotensive syndrome	• Avoid abdominal work on a noodle – consider abdominal pull ins
Oedema	• Diuretic effect which helps with reduction of oedema	• May need to urinate more frequently – plan and encourage loo breaks
Respiratory	• Pregnancy effects not compounded in water • Familiarity with hydrostatic pressure on the chest may be useful for a water birth	• Pressure on the chest or sensation of discomfort – move to shallower water
Joint instability	• Reduced stress on weight-bearing joints • Reduced impact on joints • Controlled range of movement • Reduced risk of hyperextension of joints	• Potential to hyperextend joints – observe and correct when necessary
Pelvic girdle pain	• Reduced sensation of body weight • Stress on the back and pelvis is reduced	• Pelvic girdle pain – avoid extreme range of movement around the hips and pelvis

Table 4.1	Overview of the benefits of water-based exercise in pregnancy (cont.)	
Possible diastasis	• Support for the abdominal muscles and reduced risk of diastasis	• Diastasis recti – avoid twisting and side bending activities; focus on posture throughout the session; include appropriate abdominal work
Postural changes and altered centre of gravity	• Reduced stress on the back, pelvis and other weight-bearing joints • Reduced aches and pains and low back pain	• Encourage good posture throughout • Engaging deep abdominal muscles
Thermoregulatory changes	• Water aids thermoregulation and minimises any risk of hyperthermia	• Too cool or warm may be uncomfortable – check water temperature before the session and keep moving
Breast discomfort	• Support for breasts if water under or over the bust line	• Recommend a well-fitting supportive bra • Keep arm and upper body movements smaller
Frequent urination	• Temporary relief of oedema	• Plan loo breaks • Encourage rehydration
Digestive system	• Improved digestive function	• Digestive reflux – recommend a light snack before the session; avoid positions that may increase symptoms
Carpal tunnel syndrome	• Reduced swelling and improved symptoms	• Avoid equipment or positions that put pressure on the wrists

THE PSYCHOLOGICAL BENEFITS OF WATER-BASED EXERCISE IN PREGNANCY

Water is a very soothing and relaxing environment in which to exercise and can promote a sense of calmness and wellbeing in the mother-to-be.

It has been suggested that the ability to maintain bodily control and the sense of enjoyment from activity participation has a positive mental effect (Huch & Erkkola, 1990). One study indicated that women who participated in water-based exercise during pregnancy felt they had benefited emotionally from participation (Vallim et al, 2011). Group classes have a social element which can promote socialisation and adherence to activity.

Exercising in water mimics microgravity, or very low gravity, and this can relieve feelings of discomfort from the weight of the foetus and uterus, particularly related to supine positions, exercise and breathing depth (Merati et al, 2006).

CONSIDERATIONS FOR RESUMING ACTIVITY IN THE POSTNATAL PERIOD

It is recommended that formal exercise is not restarted until after the six-week check for a normal birth and eight to ten weeks for a traumatic or lower segment Caesarean birth, and the 'all-clear' is given by medical professionals. In addition, as blood loss, or 'lochia', continues for some time after the birth it is recommended that vigorous, high-impact activities and water-based exercise is avoided until all blood loss has stopped completely. Bright red blood loss should stop after two weeks and all discharge is normally gone by about six weeks. Exercising too vigorously too soon could cause the bleeding to start again. (Note: If red blood loss is very heavy and/or continues for more than 2–3 weeks or there is accompanying fever, referral should be made to a health care professional for further investigation. These are possible signs of infection or retained placenta.)

In addition, although uterine ligaments start to return to normal very quickly, vigorous exertion in the first few days can result in severe abdominal pain so should be avoided.

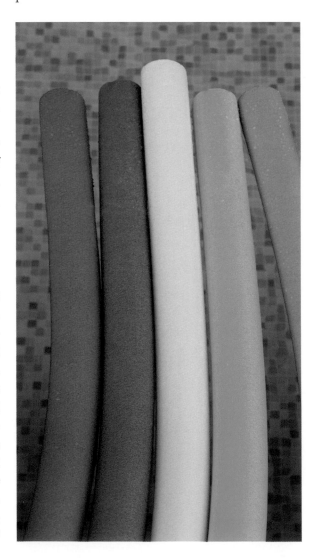

PREGNANCY AND MEDICAL CONDITIONS 5

Where pre-existing medical conditions are present, there may be significant risks for the pregnancy which make activity or exercise more hazardous for the mother-to-be. However, for many pre-existing medical conditions exercise during pregnancy is recommended to help alleviate symptoms. The following are indications of where activity may be helpful; however, full clearance to exercise must be obtained from the health care provider before starting any activity or exercise programme.

Overweight or obese

There are many risks associated with obesity in pregnancy and these include miscarriage, gestational hypertension, pre-eclampsia, pre-gestational and gestational diabetes, venous thromboembolism, pre-term delivery, urinary tract infection, asthma, sleep apnoea and gallbladder disease. For this reason it is advisable to discuss any activity plans with the health care provider.

Water-based activity may be helpful for obese pregnant women as activity can help to minimise excessive weight gain. (Note: this refers to weight gain above the recommended guidelines; activity should never be used to prevent normal or natural pregnancy weight gain.) Clearance from the main health care provider must be obtained before starting an activity programme.

Asthma (chlorine-induced)

Unless you are working in a non-chlorinated pool, water-based exercise is not recommended.

Asthma (not chlorine-induced)

Pregnancy may improve or worsen asthma symptoms, but if clearance is obtained for water-based exercise the standard pre-exercise cautions for anyone with asthma should be considered along with those for pregnancy. Water-based activity may be beneficial, provided you observe the following guidelines:

- Do not let clients exercise without their inhalers
- Do a longer warm-up of at least 10 minutes
- Alternate cardiovascular activities with muscle strength and endurance exercises
- Keep to a maximum of 4 on the intensity scale
- Perform a longer cool down − about seven minutes − and include some breathing exercises

Diabetes

For women with diabetes who are already regular exercisers, the general consensus is that they should continue to be active, although intensity may need to be lower. As with other conditions, full medical clearance must be sought.

Rheumatoid arthritis

Pregnant women with rheumatoid arthritis are unlikely to have any significant impact on the foetus as a result of the condition and being pregnant may even have a temporary beneficial effect.

If the health care provider has given clearance for exercise, some gentle activity may be beneficial, provided you follow these and any guidelines given by the health care provider:

- Perform a gradual warm-up of at least ten minutes.
- Include a good range of mobility, especially for the hips.
- Keep to low or no impact exercises, no jumping!
- Stretch carefully to avoid overstretching or extending the joints as they are affected by relaxin which can make them unstable.

Chronic fatigue conditions

Chronic fatigue conditions include chronic fatigue syndrome, myalgic encephalomyelitis, fibromyalgia or post viral fatigue syndrome. It is strongly recommended that you speak with the main health care provider before working with women with any chronic fatigue condition as energy levels may already be very low and exercise may exacerbate this. Gentle daily walking or swimming only may be appropriate during pregnancy.

Disability

If already active before pregnancy, there is usually no reason why exercise should be stopped. Instructors may wish to speak to the health care provider before starting activity, to make sure there are no potential risks or complications.

IVF pregnancy

Once pregnancy is established the exercise recommendations are the same as any other pregnancy. Due to the nature of conception, a woman may be reluctant to exercise and should always do what she feels is best for herself and the baby.

Contraindications to activity

Instructors should seek advice regarding other conditions such as multiple sclerosis, thyroid disease, post-partum thyroiditis, seizure disorders or any cardiac condition before starting an activity programme.

There are conditions where water-based exercise is definitely not suitable, including:

- Any of the Absolute Contraindications listed in the Screening section of this book
- Any of the Relative Contraindications listed in the Screening section of this book until this has been fully discussed with the woman and advice sought from health care providers if appropriate
- Any acute skin condition or infection
- Any cardiac condition affecting left ventricular function
- Extreme fear of water
- Any condition, advised by a health care provider, which may compromise the well-being of the woman or her baby or both.

This list is not exhaustive and we do strongly recommend that you consult the health care provider if a client has any pre-existing medical condition or develops one during pregnancy.

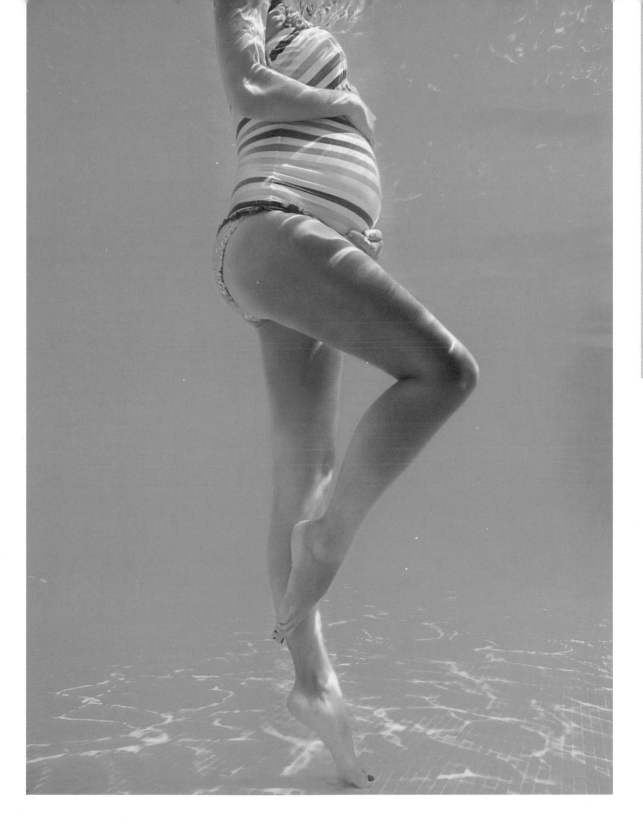

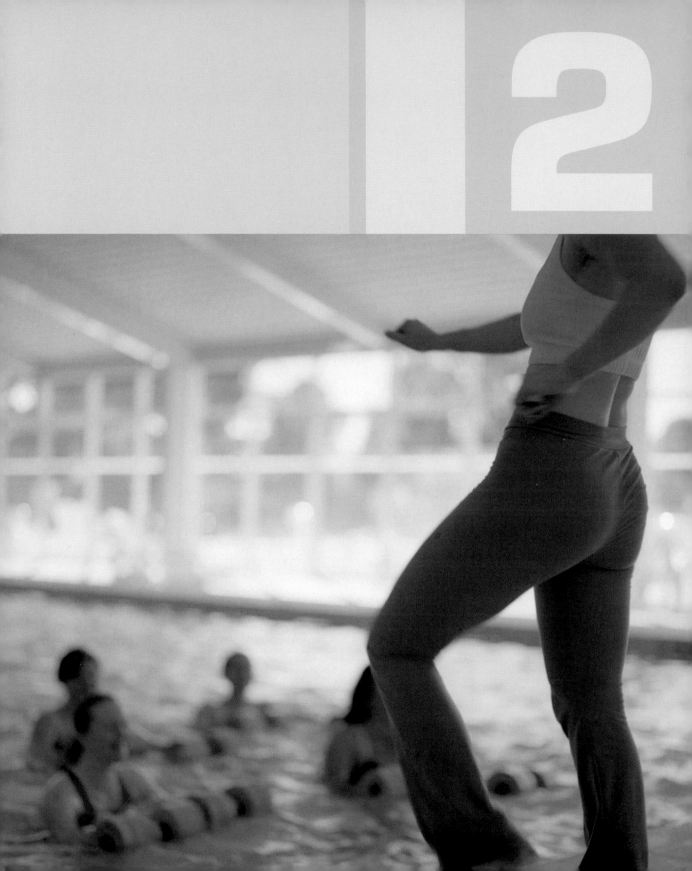

2

PART TWO

THE SKILLS

This section considers the skills an instructor needs to promote activity and support clients in adopting and adhering to a more active lifestyle. Chapter 6 covers motivating clients during pregnancy and Chapter 7 considers teaching skills and professional issues.

MOTIVATING AND SUPPORTING CLIENTS

6

MOTIVATION TO EXERCISE IN PREGNANCY

As discussed in Chapter 1, activity has many benefits for both the mother-to-be and for the foetus and many women find pregnancy acts as a trigger to improve their health behaviours, including their diet, drinking patterns and activity levels. Additionally, most women are in regular contact with at least one health care professional which makes this the ideal time to

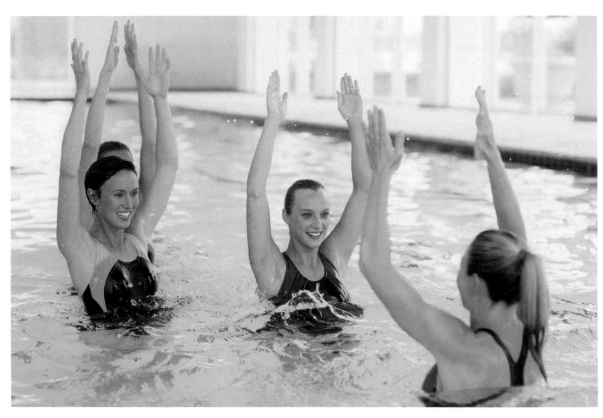

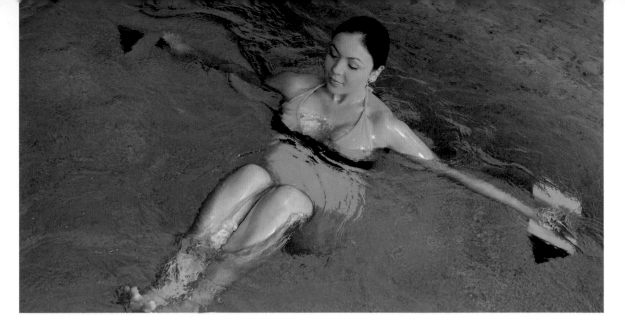

make lifestyle changes that will promote health during and after pregnancy.

However, during pregnancy, there are already many physical and mental changes occurring which can have an impact on intention to change, motivation, and on progress towards goals.

For this reason, it is important to implement small changes, focusing on the health of the mother and baby at all times. This will foster a sense of achievement and boost self-efficacy as well as having a positive impact on health.

Going from sedentary to very active is unrealistic; equally, very active women may be reluctant to 'take it easy' so changes need to be discussed and agreed if they are to be sustainable.

WHAT CAN WE DO?

As previously mentioned, a survey in 2010 found that nearly two-thirds of women (61 per cent) felt that their midwife did not have time to talk about weight management. This means instructors working with this population group are ideally placed to provide information and support on lifestyle behaviour change during pregnancy, particularly in reference to activity and exercise.

However, instructors must be aware that years of sedentary habits are not easy to overcome at any stage of life and it may be difficult for women to make lifestyle changes when they are going through the considerable physical and emotional changes of pregnancy.

Lasting behaviour change is a long-term process and the nine months of pregnancy are not really long enough to establish permanent changes, particularly with fluctuating levels of well-being, energy and motivation that are typical during this time. However, it is a good time to begin as the majority of women want to give their baby the best possible start to life and making successful changes in pregnancy is likely to promote longer adherence.

It is not possible, or practical, to discuss the many theories and models that relate to behaviour change in this book; however, it is worth mentioning that any approach you choose needs to be client-centred with their wants and needs as a focus for initiating any changes. This issue is covered in greater depth in the *Complete Guide to Behavioural Change* (Bolitho et al, 2013).

// PROFESSIONALISM

7

In this chapter we will look at the skills of a good instructor, from roles and responsibilities to teaching skills.

PROFESSIONAL ISSUES

When working with any 'specialist' population it is essential to understand the role, responsibilities and boundaries of the position.

ROLES, RESPONSIBILITIES AND LEGAL ISSUES

It is the remit of the fitness instructor to provide pregnant women with safe and effective activity advice that meets the recommended guidelines of the American Congress of Obstetricians and Gynecologists (ACOG) and, in the UK, Royal College of Obstetricians and Gynaecologists (RCOG). This is covered in qualifications on the National Occupational Standards (NOS) of the Qualification and Curriculum Framework (QCF). They may also give basic nutritional advice as recommended by the NHS and British Nutrition Foundation. Any of other advice is deemed to be outside the role and may not be covered by any recognised qualifications or insurance policies.

THE MULTI-DISCIPLINARY TEAM

Many instructors now work regularly with clients with medical conditions and this often means liaising with other health professionals in a variety of settings. Pregnancy, although not a medical condition as such, is managed by a range of health care professionals, including midwives, who make up a multi-disciplinary team. Instructors are advised to get in contact with local antenatal services to broaden their knowledge and improve team work opportunities.

If you have concerns about a pregnant or postnatal woman with whom you are working, it is your responsibility to strongly recommend she speaks to her main care provider and to defer activity until she has been seen and cleared for exercise. It is not the role or responsibility of the instructor to suggest or recommend anything other than safe and effective exercise within current recommended guidelines.

QUALIFICATIONS

Pregnant women are experiencing numerous physiological and psychological changes so any instructor working with this client group should hold the appropriate qualifications in order to give safe and effective advice about activity and exercise.

As a minimum, this would be a Level 2 Fitness Instructor qualification in Aqua, Gym or Exercise to Music PLUS a Level 3 Ante and Postnatal qualification that is recognised by the Register of Exercise Professionals. This ensures that an instructor has studied the underpinning knowledge and practical skills needed to work with this client group and meets any insurance requirements.

INSURANCE

Along with holding the appropriate qualifications, it is essential to have insurance. The two main types of insurance are Public Liability and Professional Indemnity. There are a number of companies who offer both types of insurance and who can give professional advice regarding the best options. It should go without saying that in these modern times, no instructor should be without appropriate insurance.

THE ROLE OF THE INSTRUCTOR
What makes a good instructor?

A good instructor has many qualities: empathy, knowledge, experience and awareness. They are also likely to be a good communicator, non-judgemental, a positive role model, and friendly and approachable. They also need to be able to adapt their teaching style for the poolside environment as this may require different skills to land-based sessions. These are discussed further in Section 3; however, it is useful to provide an overview here.

Teaching skills

Teaching in the poolside environment requires a number of key skills:

Instructions and explanations: Acoustics are often very poor in a pool hall so you need to ensure any instructions and explanations given are clear, simple and audible to everyone in the group. Try not to take too long to explain things as your participants are there to work out rather than listen to you and they may start to get cold! Be prepared to repeat instructions too in case people did not understand or hear you first time round.

Demonstrations: A picture is worth a thousand words so, as with your explanations, keep demonstrations clear and brief and make sure everyone can see you clearly. On poolside, this means a 'larger than life' performance at an appropriate speed so that your participant(s) can copy it in the water. It's a good idea to get the group to practise too, as this will ensure they really understand what to do and will keep them warm while they are watching your demonstration.

Teaching points: All the relevant technique and postural points that keep an exercise safe apply equally to water-based exercise – for example, joint alignment, range of movement and body position. Repeat key teaching points frequently to the group (and to specific individuals if necessary) as they are performing the exercises. This will help to keep them safe and enhance their performance overall. You will also need to consider additional teaching points to ensure that participants are utilising the water effectively. Some key points to highlight to the group are:

- Keep heels down throughout (buoyancy tends to lift the heels, which can lead to shortening of the calf muscle)
- Keep abdominals tight and 'braced' to help maintain stability (buoyancy and water resistance tend to reduce stability and balance)
- Keep shoulders down underwater (this ensures most of the body is under the water and makes the workout more effective)

- Keep arms under the water (they are needed for propulsion)
- Keep fingers together and hands cupped (this helps to make propulsive arm movements more effective)

Offering alternative exercises: It is quite likely that you will encounter a range of different fitness, skill and confidence levels within the group of women that you are teaching so there is no one-size-fits-all when it comes to exercises. Consider easier alternatives for most of the exercises that you have included so that less fit or less skilled women can keep up. Offer these as a 'more comfortable' option, rather than an easier one, so that they will be more inclined to use it. Similarly, have more challenging options available for your really fit participants so that they get an effective workout.

Observation and monitoring: You need to make sure you keep your group safe and working in the pool effectively and this can be done by using observation:

- Move around the poolside as you are teaching so that you can observe each participant and make eye contact.
- As you are moving around and observing individuals, you can quietly offer correction to technique if required. Of course, if they are performing well, praise them loudly!
- Monitor your group visually for signs of over-working, distress or cold – participants may not want to admit to feeling uncomfortable so you must be aware of the warning signs so you can offer alternatives or advice as necessary.

Warning signs: Part of observation is making sure you spot any signs of discomfort in your partici-

pants. If a woman exhibits any of the following you may need to suggest a less intense alternative, active rest or more movement if they are cold:

- Excessive shortness of breath, especially during less intense exercises
- Excessive sweating
- A dramatic change in colour – be aware of their normal colour, whether it is pale or rosy, when working out
- Inability to speak
- Wincing or grimacing – there may be muscle or joint damage
- Confusion or a lack of coordination, although some women may lack coordination in the first place!
- Shivering or 'huddled' posture

Signs to stop activity at once

If a participant complains of any of the following, stop immediately and get them out of the pool and sit or lie them down as appropriate:

- Pain in the chest
- Very sharp pain in any joint
- Severe nausea
- Feeling faint
- Severe pain in the abdomen
- Feeling very unwell in any way

Music

Aqua-natal sessions can be run either with or without music. While using music can make sessions much more fun and motivating and create a positive atmosphere, there are a number of legal issues that apply when using music that is not your own. The two main organisations you need to be aware of are PPL and PRS.

Phonographic Performance Limited (PPL)

The playing of recorded music in public requires a Phonographic Performance Limited (PPL) licence, which allows you to play music in the original, published format.

Since May 2013, a fitness centre has to pay a PPL licence fee for all classes using recorded music, whether those classes use instructors employed by the fitness centre, hired on a 'freelance' basis by the centre, or are taught by individual instructors hiring out the facilities in that centre. In addition, since May 2013, a fitness instructor has to ensure they pay a PPL licence fee (based on a fee per class basis) if they are teaching and using recorded music in premises other than fitness centres – for example, hired halls and offices.

The only exceptions to this may be if the event is wholly for charity, not profit, or at a private event such as a birthday party. PPL do 'mystery shopper' visits so if you are going to play any music that is not your own original composition and recording during sessions you must ensure the appropriate licence is in place or face a heavy fine or even imprisonment.

For information on obtaining a licence contact PPL direct on: Telephone: 020 7534 1000; Website: www.ppluk.com

Note: A PPL licence does not allow you to make and then play compilations or to transfer recordings onto a disc, laptop or other playing device for use in public.

There are various companies that supply both a PPL Licence and prepared music with speed (beats per minute) details given. Subscribers pay a set fee per month or year for the licence and can choose from a variety of levels of membership that include an allocation of music recordings.

There are also various companies that offer PPL licence-free recordings. These are not by the original artist or group, but have been re-recorded to avoid having to pay for the licence.

Performing Right Society (PRS)

PRS is a not-for-profit organisation that collects licence fees from music users and distributes these in the form of royalties to the writers/publishers of music in the UK and internationally. The Copyright Designs and Patents Act 1988 requires you to have permission from the writer/composer of any music you wish to play in public; however, the logistics of this would be very complicated so the Performing Right Society (PRS) Music Licence gives you the legal permission to do this more simply.

Any location or premises, outside of home, where music is played will need a PRS Music Licence. This includes leisure centres, church halls and private health clubs. The owner/proprietor of the premises is normally responsible for obtaining a PRS Music Licence for the public performance of copyright music.

As with the PPL licence, there are legal implications if you are caught without a licence. Due to licensing requirements, many venues and centres hold a PRS Music Licence so check in advance if this is the case. There are various tariffs and information can be obtained from PRS on: Telephone: 0800 068 4828; Website: www.mcps-prs-alliance.co.uk

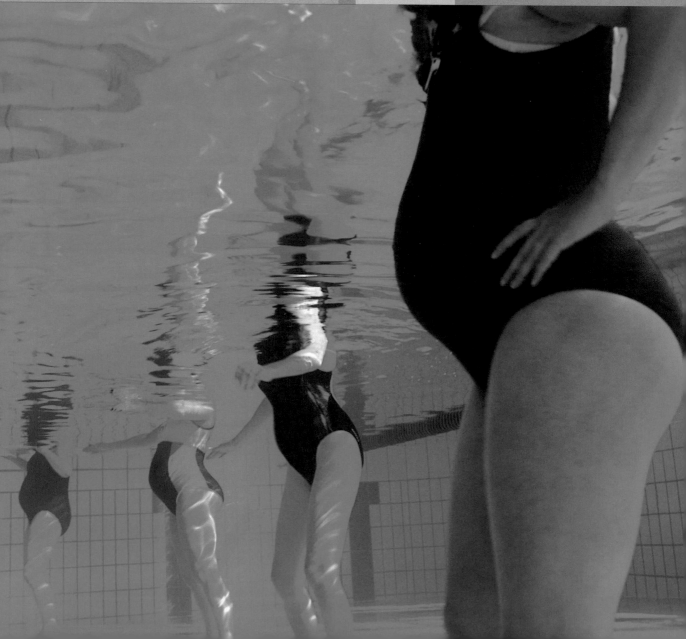

3

PART **THREE**

PRACTICAL APPLICATION

This section focuses on the practical application of water-based exercise for pregnant and postnatal women. Chapter 8 includes information on screening and risk stratification using guidelines set out by the American Congress of Obstetricians and Gynecologists and the UK's Royal College of Obstetricians and Gynaecologists. However, these guidelines are updated from time to time so instructors must check on a regular basis to ensure they are working to the latest recommendations. Chapter 9 looks at planning and delivering water-based activity sessions.

Chapters 10 and 11 list a wide range of exercises suitable for pre- and postnatal water-based exercise sessions and Chapter 12 includes some sample classes.

SCREENING AND RISK STRATIFICATION

SCREENING

It is essential to screen all pregnant women prior to starting activity or exercise, or with regular exercisers when they tell you they are pregnant. Also re-screen at regular intervals during the pregnancy as their condition may change. Postnatal women must be screened on return to exercise and it is recommended that they are re-screened on a regular basis until they have fully returned to normal, usually six months post delivery.

INITIAL PRE-ACTIVITY SCREENING

Pre-activity screening is an important part of the preparation for activity and all pregnant women must complete a PAR-Q prior to participation. This should be specific to pregnancy and it may be necessary to consult with the primary care giver if there are any areas of concern. An example of a pre-exercise screening form for pregnant women is the PAR-MedX for Pregnancy which is available to download and use in the original format from the Canadian Society of Exercise Physiologists at www.csep.ca.

A woman who answers 'no' to all questions should be suitable for participation without further clearance, but if she answers 'yes' to one or more questions she must be referred to her GP or midwife for clearance before participation. If you are in any doubt, you must consult her health care professional, an exercise referral instructor or your manager for advice prior to including the participant in any activity.

PRE-SESSION SCREENING

It is likely that the health status of pregnant women will change from time to time so it is important to do a verbal and visual screen before each session. This can be done with the group, but you do need to offer privacy for women who may want to tell you of a more personal change in their health status. Not everyone wants to announce to the whole group that they have developed piles, or stress incontinence!

Both before a session and during it, a visual screen can be used to check facial colour, posture, swelling, gait, and general demeanour, so that anything unusual or worrying can be discussed quietly with the participant.

Be aware that a pregnant woman is carrying a baby which can be very stressful, and while appropriate exercise and activity is usually beneficial and unlikely to present a risk to the foetus, she may be cautious 'just in case'. If exercise is going to cause anxiety or worry it is better that she does not participate until she feels ready. You can recommend gentle walking or swimming, but if she wants to sit in front of daytime telly with her feet up then that is fine! Just reassure her that she can come back to exercise after the birth.

CONTRAINDICATIONS AND CAUTIONS TO EXERCISE IN PREGNANCY

The American College (Congress) of Obstetricians and Gynecologists publish recommendations and guidelines for exercise during the pre- and postnatal periods including a comprehensive list of contraindications (ACOG, 2009). These are rein-forced by the Royal College of Obstetricians and Gynaecologists in the UK (RCOG, 2006). The current ACOG recommendations were published in January 2002 and revised in 2009; however, new recommendations may be published at any time and it is advised that instructors check the ACOG website regularly for information.

Contraindications to activity

There are conditions or indications which make activity during pregnancy contraindicated. These should be followed at all times to avoid any risk to the mother or foetus from inappropriate activity.

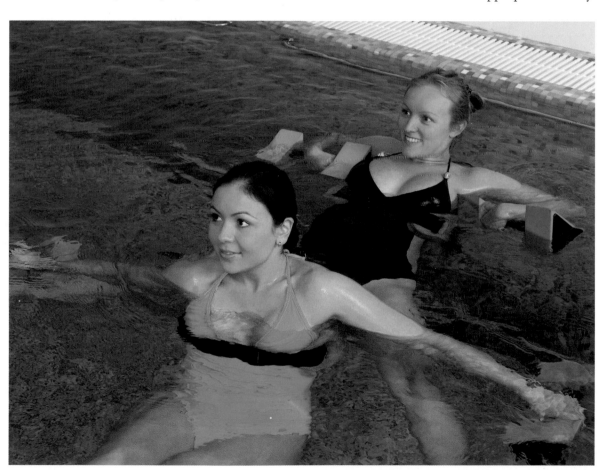

Absolute contraindications to activity – pregnancy

There are a number of absolute contraindications to exercise during pregnancy set out by both ACOG and RCOG. These are listed in the box below, and must be strictly followed.

Absolute contraindications to exercise – general

As well as the conditions that may occur during pregnancy, discussed earlier, there are cautions and contraindications to participation in exercise that apply to anyone, pregnant or not.

Absolute contraindications in pregnancy

- Haemodynamically significant heart disease
- Restrictive lung disease
- Incompetent cervix/cerclage (a stitch in the cervix to help it remain closed)*
- Multiple gestation at risk for premature labour
- Persistent 2nd or 3rd trimester bleeding
- Placenta praevia after 26 weeks gestation
- Premature labour during the current pregnancy
- Ruptured membranes
- Pregnancy induced hypertension or pre-eclampsia

* Note that some consultants are happy to allow women who have a cerclage (also known as a cervical stitch) in situ as a result of an incompetent cervix to participate in activity; however, permission must be sought from the consultant.

Absolute contraindications to activity

- Heart or circulation problems
- New or uncontrolled diabetes
- New or uncontrolled tachycardia (RHR>100)
- Blood pressure levels over 180/100 (either figure)
- Ventricular or aortic aneurysm
- Stroke or transient ischaemic attack
- New or uncontrolled arrhythmias
- Any acute infection or disease
- An unexplained asthma attack or excessive shortness of breath on mild exertion
- A flare up of arthritis
- Vomiting or diarrhoea
- Fever, flu, severe cold or a viral infection or feeling unusually unwell
- Any injury or increased or new pain in any joint

If your participants have any of the conditions listed in the box above or develop them during pregnancy, whether they are linked to the pregnancy or not, they should not participate in exercise.

Remember, if there's doubt, they're out.

Relative contraindications to activity in pregnancy

In addition to the absolute contraindications to exercise in pregnancy and generally, there are a number of relative contraindications to exercise including those listed in the boxes. However, exercise may still be undertaken if full medical clearance is obtained from the doctor or midwife before starting or returning to activity.

SIGNS TO STOP EXERCISE IN PREGNANCY

There are also a number of warning signs that indicate immediate cessation of an exercise session or stopping all exercise during pregnancy (ACOG, 2009; RCOG, 2006). These include but are not limited to:

- Vaginal bleeding
- Chest pain
- Oedema of hands and/or ankles
- Calf pain or swelling (need to rule out thrombophlebitis)
- Dyspnoea (breathing problems) before exertion
- Dizziness
- Headache
- Preterm labour
- Decreased foetal movement
- Amniotic fluid leakage
- Muscle weakness

The ACOG recommendations (ACOG, 2002) also offer guidelines for sports and recreational activities which include caution against participation in contact sports or activities with an increased risk of falling or of abdominal trauma such as riding, gymnastics or skiing (downhill), and avoidance of scuba diving due to an increased risk of decompression sickness in the foetus. Activity at altitudes of more than 2500 m (6000 ft) should also be avoided.

For the majority of pregnant women, activity will be a welcome part of their routine and provided none of the above contraindications is present, participation in appropriate exercise is strongly recommended.

Relative contraindications in pregnancy

- Severe anaemia
- Unevaluated maternal cardiac arrhythmia
- Chronic bronchitis
- Poorly controlled type 1 diabetes
- Intrauterine growth restriction in current pregnancy
- Poorly controlled hypertension
- Poorly controlled seizure disorder
- Poorly controlled thyroid disease
- Orthopaedic limitations
- Extreme morbid obesity
- Extreme underweight (body mass index <12)
- History of extremely sedentary lifestyle
- Heavy smoker
- Acute illness or infection

PLANNING AND DELIVERING WATER-BASED EXERCISE

9

PRE-SESSION CONSIDERATIONS

In addition to pre-exercise screening, discussed in Chapter 8, there are other things to consider when working in the pool environment. It is good practice to undertake a full risk assessment of the environment when assessing the suitability of a pool for prenatal sessions, and then to review it regularly.

ACCESS IN AND OUT OF THE POOL

The area around the pool is obviously likely to be wet and therefore potentially slippery. The entry of participants in and out of the pool needs to be supervised. Make sure they are not rushing and that they do use entry steps and hand rails, if available. If participants need to get out of the pool during the session for a toilet break, reinforce the advice to use hand rails where available and not to rush, since they will be wet which increases the potential for slipping. They will also need to re-adjust to their increased weight and centre of gravity when they are no longer buoyant.

Jumping or diving into the water should always be discouraged as this may lead to abdominal trauma or affect lax joints at any stage of pregnancy.

POOLSIDE SAFETY

As the instructor, when teaching on poolside consider appropriate footwear and use of mats to minimise slippage and maximise shock absorption, especially when performing high impact activities and jumping. Slipping and falling on poolside can be painful, and embarrassing!

WATER TEMPERATURE

As already mentioned, about 30 degrees Celsius is ideal for prenatal aqua sessions. The surrounding air should be about 1 degree Celsius higher for comfort when participants exit the pool. Cooler water could leave participants feeling chilled, while warmer water may lead to vasodilation, hypotension, fainting and fatigue. Hospital hydrotherapy pools are appropriate for controlled and static rehabilitation activities, but may be too warm for more dynamic and continuous exercise usually performed in prenatal aqua sessions.

WATER DEPTH

As already stated, the ideal depth for a water-based prenatal exercise session is anywhere between chest and shoulders, keeping the arms underwater. At the xiphisternum, the abdominal corset is supported, but the upper body may remain cool. As the water reaches the shoulders, the upper body stays warmer and arms can be used effectively under the water for any propulsion that may be required; however, buoyancy increases and this will challenge stability and balance. In addition, if breasts are tender or sore they may be more comfortable under the water and fully supported by the buoyancy, or they may be better out of the water without hydrostatic pressure around them.

While you need to check with the participants what depth is most comfortable for them, the minimum depth should be at the xiphisternum.

As previously discussed, you need to remember that even if the pool is all one depth, people of different heights will experience different levels of buoyancy and resistance. Shorter individuals will be more deeply submerged and potentially more buoyant. Taller people will experience less buoyancy and resistance but more impact.

TOILET FACILITIES

Ensure there are sufficient, accessible toilet facilities available for those inevitable loo breaks. If participants get out of the pool to use the facilities, remind them to use the entry steps and take care on the wet, slippery poolside. Use hand rails where available and walk rather than run.

ELECTRICAL EQUIPMENT

If using a music system on poolside, ensure it has a current safety certificate (PAT) and, if it is mains-powered, is used in conjunction with a circuit breaker. If it is a battery-powered system, make sure you have a spare set of batteries available. With all equipment, place it as far away from the water as possible, including the potential 'splash' zone.

SESSION STRUCTURE AND CONTENT

The emphasis of a typical aqua-natal training session should be on movement quality and posture. Ideally, it will consist of a range of dynamic exercises to promote mobility and circulation, together with specific muscular strength and endurance exercises with or without equipment. These muscular strength and endurance exercises should be targeted at areas of the body that may be particularly affected by the woman's changing body shape and also those muscles that will be involved in childcare activities once the baby is born.

The session should always begin with a warm-up to prepare the whole body for the planned activities and it should finish with a cool down to return the body to its pre-exercise state and promote a feeling of relaxation and well-being.

THE INITIAL WELCOME AND INTRODUCTION

The welcome participants receive as they come into the class has a great impact on how they think they will enjoy it. Wherever you greet participants, in reception, or by poolside, welcoming previous participants back warmly, asking how they are, and taking time to introduce yourself to newcomers and ask about their experience of aqua exercise is a good way to start the class. You can also do a quick individual verbal screen to check current health status and any new contraindications and a visual screen of the group to spot anything you may want to discuss.

This may also be an appropriate time to inform participants of your professional qualifications and experience, in order to reassure them and promote confidence in your abilities.

THE WARM-UP

Due to the hydrostatic pressure and buoyancy of water, your warm-up may be slightly quicker than on land; however, it does need to be gradual and longer than for a non-pregnant group of exercisers. The components of the warm-up remain the same; include mobilising and pulse raising activities in order to prepare bones, joints and the circulatory system. Pre-stretching may also be necessary for key muscles such as gastrocnemius and pectoralis. Keep moves as big and dynamic as is comfortable to ensure that the individuals stay warm, but be aware of breast discomfort with arm movements, and lower back or hip discomfort which may be a sign of dysfunction in the pelvis. The total warm-up should take approximately eight to ten minutes depending on the fitness level and experience of the group.

Mobility

Joints need to be taken through a full, comfortable range to promote secretion of synovial fluid and warm the connective tissues and structures at each joint. Resistance of the water slows moves down, and buoyancy supports limbs, so you can start with big, full-range moves straight away. Most joints can be mobilised effectively in combination with pulse raising in order to keep the group moving and warm.

Pulse raising

Working muscles need a greater delivery of oxygen to maintain the workload in the main workout and this is achieved by gradually raising the pulse to increase blood flow to the muscles. Buoyancy cushions joints, so if comfortable, allow participants to add some 'spring' to their movements to facilitate pulse raising and maintain warmth.

It is useful to include less intense versions of the exercises and/or lower impact activities for anyone less fit or experiencing some of the discomforts of pregnancy, or who is just plain tired.

Pre-stretching

It is important to consider some of the postural changes of pregnancy when deciding which stretches to include at the beginning of the session. Muscles tending to be short and/or tight in pregnancy include pectorals, hip flexors, hamstrings and calf muscles. For this reason, it is appropriate to include stretches for these muscle groups to start to encourage full range of movement in these areas. Joints may be lax and balance may be challenged by the altered body shape and the buoyancy of the water, so it may be advisable to perform static, supported stretches using floats or at the poolside to assist stability. Muscles that may be lengthened in pregnancy include trapezius and the abdominals including obliques, so it may be appropriate to omit stretches for these areas to avoid lengthening them further. However, dynamic movements will loosen off any tension that may be present. Keep the group moving in between static stretches to keep them warm.

Rewarming

After stretching make sure your participants are warm enough to start the main workout. The activities included here can be the same as for pulse raising with some increased impact, more travel and larger moves incorporated if participants are comfortable to do so. This can be quite a short component, approximately 4 minutes, because:

a) hydrostatic pressure is helping blood flow more efficiently, and

b) intensity should not have dropped much in the pre-stretching component due to keeping the group moving and warm in between stretches.

MAIN WORKOUT

Your main workout can be organised in a number of ways, depending on the aims of the session and the group. Not all your participants will be skilled and experienced, so you may need to demonstrate some exercises. If you have included new or complex exercises, you should demonstrate these too. Just remember:

- Aim to include the demonstrations within your warm-up and 're-warming' so that you can move smoothly into the main workout without having to stop and show the exercises once everyone is warmed up and raring to go
- Keep demonstrations clear and brief
- Keep the group moving and warm while you are demonstrating. Get them to rehearse the exercise or a similar movement
- Let the group practise once you have demonstrated. This will enhance self-efficacy and promote autonomy.

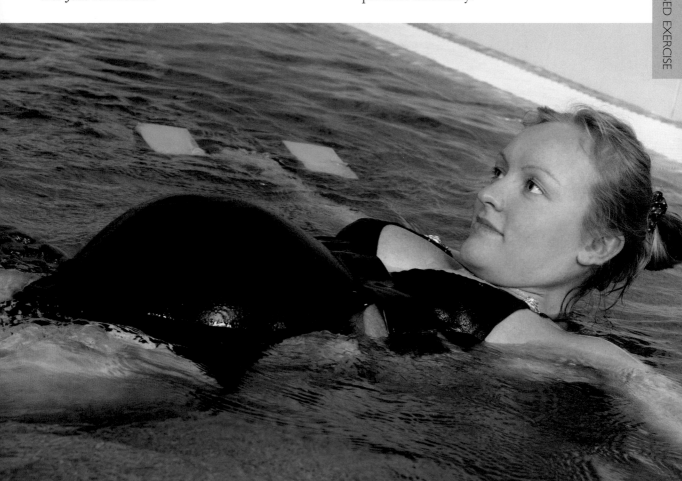

Total time for the main component should be around 20 minutes, which falls well within current ACOG and RCOG guidelines. Your session could be one of the following formats:

1. Exercise to music

- Aerobic exercises
- Aerobic and muscle toning exercises to music

This style of class could be 'choreographed' to music or the activities could be performed in sequence using the music to pace the movements.

2. Circuit style

- The exercise stations could be in a circle around the pool edge
- The exercise stations could be in small groups at each corner of the pool
- The group could be split in half, with one half of the group doing one exercise, and the other half of the group doing a different exercise

Aerobic activities

When planning cardiovascular activities, remember to keep speed of movement moderate and allow time for changes of direction because of changes in the woman's centre of gravity and the influences of frontal resistance and eddy drag. As already stated, take care with range of movement throughout.

Any 'choreography' or movement sequences should be relatively short and simple so that they can be easily followed. When changing direction, consider performing a movement 'on the spot' so that participants have time to transition safely whilst maintaining good technique and posture; for example, after jogging or walking forward, perform some knee lifts or low leg kicks on the spot before jogging back. This also allows for any eddy drag effects to disperse. Performing more repetitions of each move – for example, four steps to the side rather than two; or eight squats rather than four – will also allow participants to perform each activity more effectively and transition more safely. It will also allow more time to 'cue' the next activity well in advance.

Muscular toning activities

When planning strength and endurance work, as with stretches, consider which muscles are affected by the growing pregnancy and may need strengthening – good examples include:

- Deep abdominal muscles (transverse abdominals)
- Trapezius
- Gluteals
- Pelvic floor

It is also worthwhile including muscles that will be involved in childcare activities, such as:

- Pectorals and triceps for buggy pushing
- Quadriceps, gluteals and hamstrings for lifting baby and baby's stuff
- Trapezius and biceps for lifting and carrying

Throughout the workout, as already mentioned, take care with range of movement for all activities. Although the buoyancy and resistance of the water help to support limbs the mother may still be able to lock out knees and elbows more easily and turn her ankles due to joint laxity, so observe participants carefully to make sure they are not hyperextending any joints. Also take care with speed of movement and transitions to ensure that participants are able to maintain good posture and form when moving and changing direction.

COOLING DOWN

Pulse lowering

The aim of the cool down section is to return the heart and breathing rates to a steady pre-exercise state. This is achieved by reducing the intensity and impact or by reversing the moves from the pulse raising section. Again, due to the water properties, this section can be a little quicker than on land, approximately 3–4 minutes, but it still needs to be smooth and very gradual. Take time to chat to your participants so you can tell from their breathing that they are getting back to a comfortable state. Breathing may still be a bit heavier than normal, but individuals should be able to talk freely. Most importantly, they should still feel warm.

Post-workout stretches

All muscles worked in the session should be stretched during the cool down. However, prolonged (developmental) stretching, aimed at improving flexibility, is not appropriate due to the effects of relaxin on the joints and the risk of stretching ligaments and tendons. Participants could also get very cold and uncomfortable during this time. Shorter hold stretches, aimed at maintaining flexibility, incorporating some movement in between as in the warm-up, are the best way to go. These static stretches should be done using the pool wall, the lane marker or a float for support. Offer alternatives for the more or less flexible participants and check too that individuals are not getting cold.

Overall this final section of the class should take about 5–7 minutes, including a short relaxation section.

However any relaxant needs to be active to ensure participants stay warm.

AND AFTER THE SESSION

As part of ongoing professional development as fitness or health professionals, it is important to obtain and act on feedback from our participants. Take time at the end of the session to ask for feedback, find out what they liked and what they didn't and how they felt during and after the session – it will help with the planning and development of sessions that are motivating and enjoyable and keep classes well attended. It may also be another good opportunity for information-giving.

Consider having this feedback session over a warm drink and a snack once participants are dry and changed. This will stop them getting cold while standing around in the pool or dripping wet on poolside and the warm drink is necessary to counter any potential drop in blood sugar levels and blood pressure after exercise.

Blood glucose levels decrease more rapidly in pregnant women when exercising and remain lower after exercise as well, making hypoglycaemia more likely. It is well worth advising pregnant women to have a light, good quality carbohydrate snack about one hour prior to exercise, in addition to a post-exercise drink and snack.

INTENSITY

It is important to monitor intensity during the session and one of the simplest and most effective ways of doing this is to use a rating of perceived exertion scale. There are two well evidenced versions of this scale, both shown below. The full Borg scale runs from 6–20 while the modified CR10 scale runs from 0–10 (Borg, 1970, 1982). For most people the 0–10 is the easiest to understand and use, but whichever you choose, ensure you explain it well and use it regularly. You could prepare a large chart that you can hold up during the session as a visual aid.

The intensity of the workout needs to be at a level that promotes health benefits, but does not compromise safety of mother or baby.

By the end of the warm-up, intensity should be no more than 3–4 on the chart below. The main workout should not exceed 6 although for less fit participants it may be more appropriate to keep them at around 4, as long as they stay warm. The cool down should gradually reduce intensity back to around 2 or 1.

Table 9.1	Rating of Perceived Exertion Scale			
Full Borg 6–20 scale		**Comments**	**Modified CR 10 scale**	
No exertion at all	6	Warm-up/Cool down zone	Nothing at all	0
Extremely light	7		Very very weak	0.5
	8			
Very light	9		Very weak	1
	10		Weak	2
Light	11		Moderate	3
	12	Aerobic zone	Somewhat hard	4
Somewhat hard	13			5
	14		Hard	6
Hard (heavy)	15			7
	16	Intervals – anaerobic zone	Very hard	8
Very hard	17			
	18			9
Extremely hard	19		Very very hard	
Max exertion	20			10

(Adapted from Borg, 1982)

PRENATAL EXERCISES

10

This chapter contains a range of exercises suitable for an antenatal class. The warm-up exercises can also be used as cardiovascular activities in the main section or as pulse lowering activities. The intensity will need to be adapted for each component.

Purpose
To teach and reinforce good posture at the start.

Start position and instructions
Standing in water at chest depth, with feet about hip width apart or with one foot about one pace in front of the other. Whichever position the feet are in, weight should be evenly distributed through both legs.

Teaching points
- Shoulders rolled back and down, head lifted, neck long and chin tucked in.
- Abdominal muscles pulled in, gluteal muscles tightened slightly to tuck the pelvis and coccyx ('tailbone') under. This should give the feeling of pulling the baby-bump upwards and inwards, whilst lifting the ribcage.

WARM-UP EXERCISES
PREPARATION

Ex 10.1 Posture check

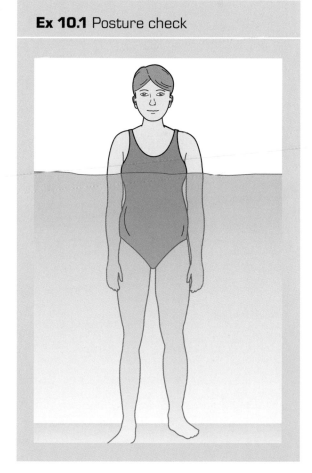

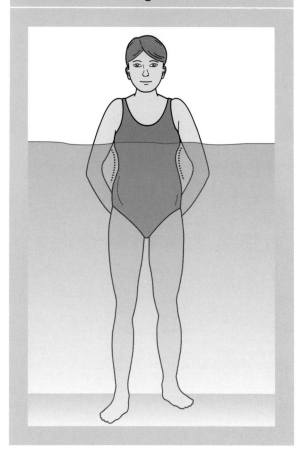

Ex 10.2 Breathing exercise

Purpose

To bring awareness to breathing and help to develop the ability to breathe fully and deeply.

Start position and instructions

A normal breathing pattern should be maintained throughout the aqua-natal session. Breath holding should be avoided and participants should be encouraged to breathe normally, especially when stretching or concentrating during more strenuous activities. Try some deeper breaths at the very start and at the end of the session in any comfortable position.

Teaching points

- Avoid holding the breath.
- Breathe out during the effort/exertion phase of any exercise and inhale on the relaxation/release phase of the exercise.

Ex 10.3 Pelvic floor contractions

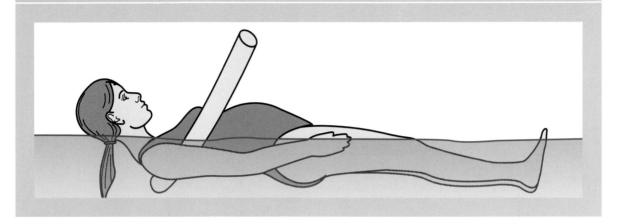

Purpose

To locate and strengthen the pelvic floor muscles. This exercise could be done in the cool down section of the session.

Start position and instructions

Stand with feet about hip width apart or with one foot about one pace in front of the other
OR
Sitting, balanced on a noodle shaped float
OR
Floating on back with noodle shaped float under the shoulders for support

Slow contractions:

- Start back or front, whatever is more natural/easier for participant
- Draw up and close back passage, draw up and close front passage
- Squeeze and lift up inside the body/vagina
- Keep breathing and hold for 6–10 seconds and then let go slowly
- You should, with practice, over time be able to increase the length of hold up to 10 seconds as the muscles become stronger

- Aim for 4–10 reps.

Fast contractions:

- Draw up and close back passage, draw up and close front passage
- Squeeze and lift up quickly inside body/vagina
- Keep breathing and hold very briefly for approx 1 second and then let go slowly
- Aim for 4–10 reps.

Teaching points

- Avoid holding the breath, tightening abdominal muscles and clenching the buttocks whilst locating and contracting the pelvic floor.
- Consider lowering eyes downwards or closing eyes to avoid looking at others and feeling self conscious.

Alternatives

- Easy: Fewer contractions or just hold for as long as is comfortable.
- Easy: If floating on the back is difficult, try using a second noodle under the hips or lower back.

PULSE RAISING/CARDIOVASCULAR EXERCISES

Ex 10.4 Jogging or walking on the spot

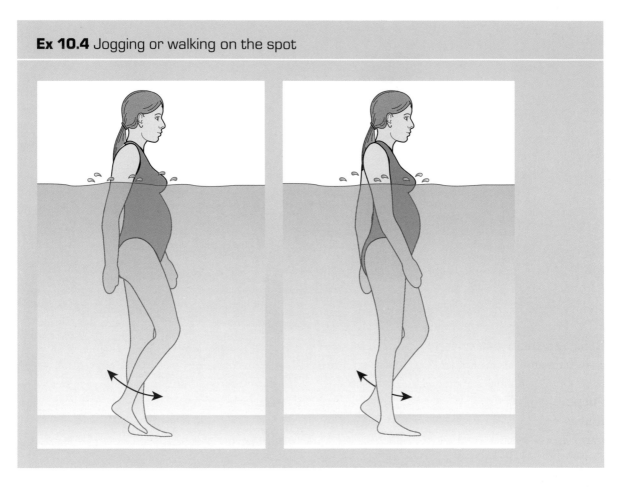

Note: Remember that walking on the spot will not maintain body temperature as efficiently as a light jog.

Purpose
This is a pulse raising activity and will help to warm up the body.

Start position and instructions
Standing in water at chest depth, with knees loose and joints not locked. Lift legs into a march or jog.

Teaching points
Shoulders under the water, hips and baby-bump facing forward. Heels down.

Alternatives
- Easy: Adjust the speed of the jog/march, smaller march on the spot.
- Harder: Higher knees.

Ex 10.5 Walking or jogging forwards and backwards

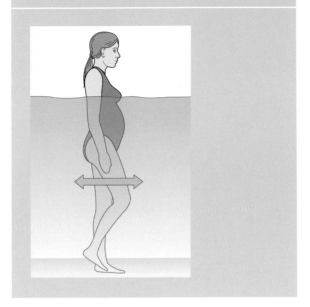

Ex 10.6 Walking or jogging around the pool

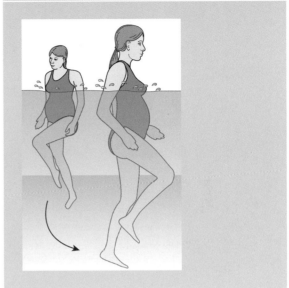

Note: Remember that walking will not maintain body temperature as efficiently as a light jog.

Purpose
This is a pulse raising activity and will help to warm up the body.

Start position and instructions
Standing in water at chest depth, with knees loose and joints not locked. Travel forwards and backwards.

Teaching points
Shoulders under water, hips and baby-bump facing forward. Heels down.

Alternatives
* Easy: Stay on the spot and jog/march.
* Harder: Lift knees higher, travel further.

Purpose
This is a pulse raising activity to warm the body further.

Start position and instructions
Standing in water at chest depth, with knees loose and joints not locked. Lift legs into a march or jog and travel around the pool in a circle.

Teaching points
Shoulders under water, hips and baby-bump facing forward. Heels down. Slower participants jog on the inside, faster participants on the outside of the circle.

Alternatives
* Easy: March on the spot.
* Easy: March forward and back.
* Harder: Higher knees.

Ex 10.7 'Pony' walking

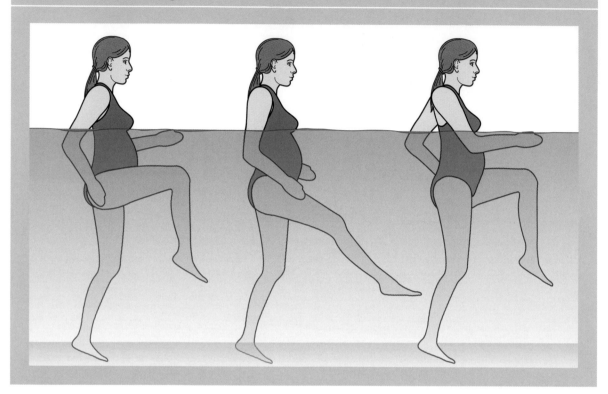

Purpose
To warm up the body.

Start position and instructions
Standing in water at chest depth, with knees loose and joints not locked. Raise the knee to a comfortable height and then straighten the leg out in front before lowering the foot to the pool floor. Change legs and repeat the action whilst moving forwards.

Teaching points
- Avoid leaning forwards.
- Keep hips level and baby-bump facing forwards.

Alternatives
- Easy: Lower knee raise.
- Harder: Try with arms behind back to challenge balance further.

Ex 10.8 Knee lifts

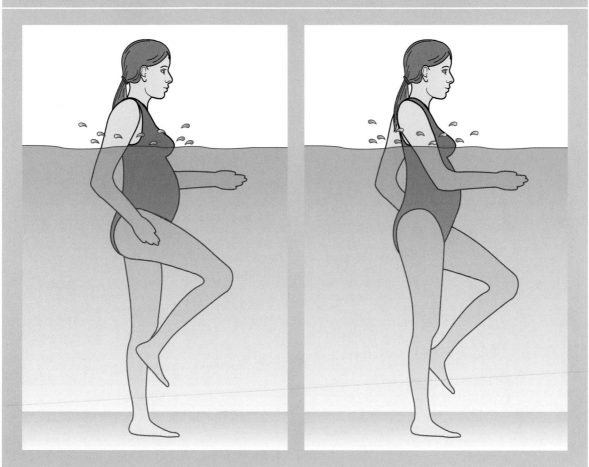

Purpose
Pulse raising combined with hip and knee mobility.

Start position and instructions
Standing in water at chest depth, with knees loose and joints not locked. Lift knee up towards hip level, then change legs.

Teaching points
Hips, knees and toes all in line. Keep heels down and shoulders under the water.

Alternatives
- Easy: Smaller moves.
- Harder: Bigger moves.
- Harder: Add a spring.
- If the baby-bump is large, reduce height of knee lift or take knee slightly out to the side.

Ex 10.9 Leg curls

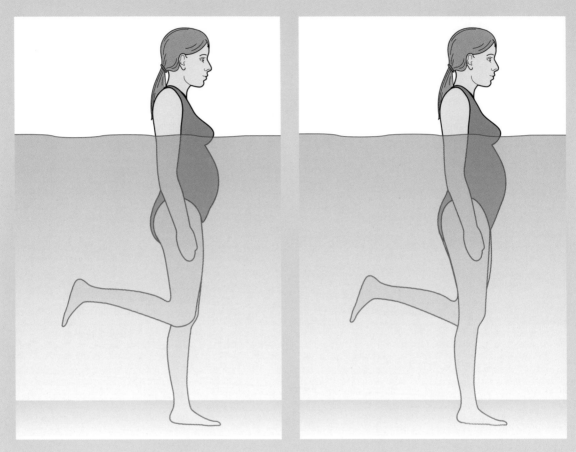

Purpose
Pulse raising and knee mobility.

Start position and instructions
Standing in water at chest depth, with knees loose and joints not locked. Lift heel up towards backside, then change legs.

Teaching points
- Keep heels down and shoulders under the water.
- Keep the baby-bump pulled in and hips facing forwards.

Alternatives
- Easy: Smaller curl.
- Easy: Jog.
- Harder: Add a spring as legs change.

Ex 10.10 Side steps

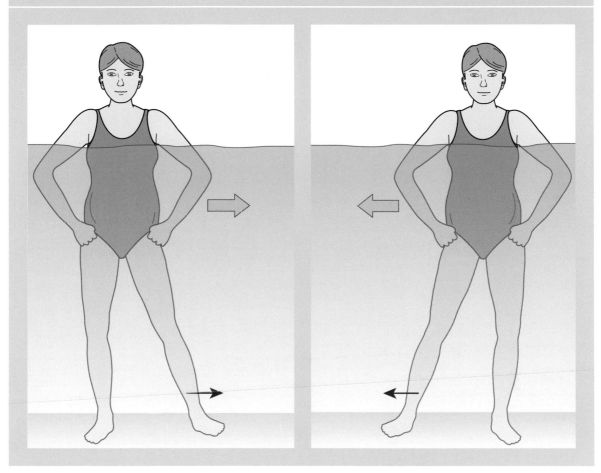

Purpose
Pulse raising/aerobic.

Start position and instructions
Standing in water at chest depth, with knees loose and joints not locked. Facing forwards, take a step to the side, then back to the other side.

Teaching points
Shoulders under the water, brace abdominals. Hips forward, heels down. Arms pull across body opposite to direction of travel. Fingers together, hands cupped.

Alternatives
* Easy: Narrower side steps.
* Easy: Turn and walk in the direction of the side steps.
* Harder: Wider step with deeper knee bends (care to avoid pelvic discomfort).

Ex 10.11 Imaginary skipping

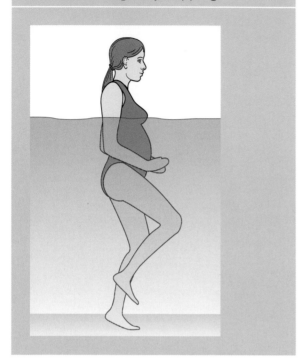

Purpose
Pulse raising.

Start position and instruction
- Standing in water at chest depth, with knees loose and joints not locked.
- Perform a skipping movement and use the wrists as if using a rope.

Teaching points
Shoulders under the water, hips and baby-bump facing forward. Heels down. Keep arms underwater and use an imaginary skipping rope.

Alternatives
- Easy: Walk or jog on the spot.
- Harder: Lift legs higher, add more spring.

MOBILITY EXERCISES

Ex 10.12 Biceps curls

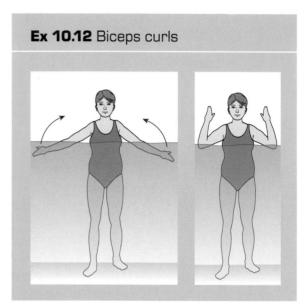

Purpose
Elbow joint mobility. Best performed with some jogging to prevent participants getting cold.

Start position and instructions
Standing in water at chest depth, with knees loose and joints not locked. Bend arms at elbows and raise up towards shoulders.

Teaching points
Keep elbows tucked in to the sides of the body and keep arms underwater throughout the movement.

Alternatives
- Easy: One arm at a time. Open fingers or slice the hands.
- Harder: Keep fingers closed.

Ex 10.13 Breaststroke arms

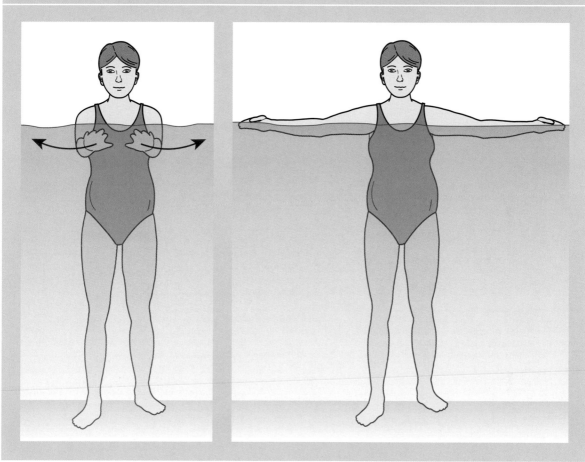

Purpose
Shoulder mobility and a dynamic stretch for pectorals.

Start position and instructions
Standing in water at chest depth, with knees loose and joints not locked and feet hip width apart or with one foot about one pace in front of the other. Whichever position the feet are in, weight should be evenly distributed through both legs. Start with arms together under the water in front of the body and move them apart in a breaststroke style.

Teaching points
Shoulders under the water, brace abdominals. Hips forward, heels down. Fingers together.

Alternatives
- Easy: Slice hands through the water with a flat hand.
- Easy: Open the fingers.

Ex 10.14 Forward arm pushes

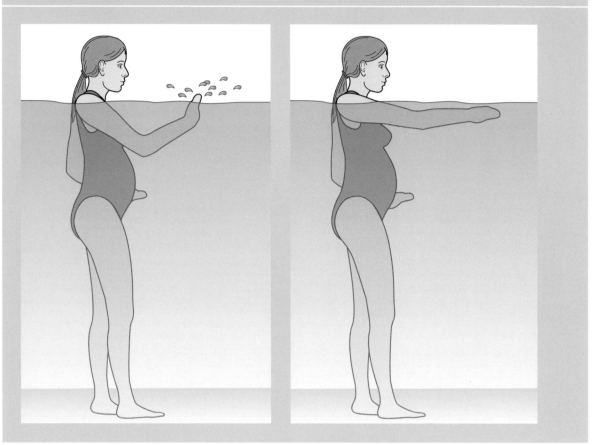

Purpose
Shoulder and elbow mobility.

Start position and instructions
Standing in water at chest depth, with knees loose and joints not locked and feet hip width apart or with one foot about one pace in front of the other. Whichever position the feet are in, weight should be evenly distributed through both legs. Start with arms just under the water surface, palms facing forward. Push one arm forward to straighten the elbow. Swap arms and repeat.

Teaching points
Shoulders under the water, brace abdominals. Hips and baby-bump facing forward, heels down. Fingers together.

Alternatives
- Easy: Slice hands through the water.
- Easy: Open the fingers.
- Harder: Speed up the movement or push both arms forward together instead of alternating the arms.

Ex 10.15 Forward arm sweeps

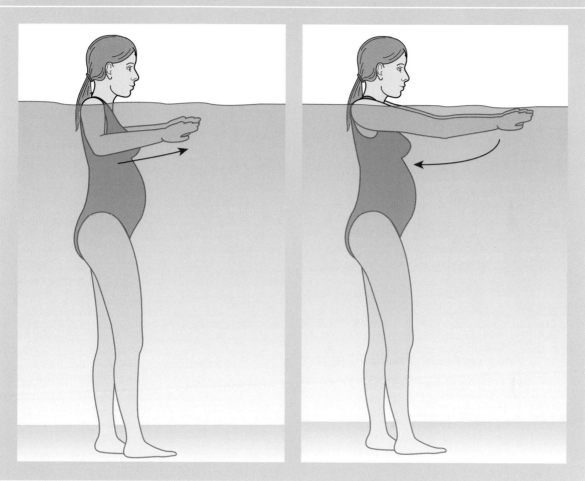

Purpose
Shoulder mobility and a dynamic stretch for pectorals and trapezius.

Start position and instructions
Standing in water at chest depth, with knees loose and joints not locked and feet hip width apart or with one foot about one pace in front of the other. Whichever position the feet are in, weight should be evenly distributed through both legs.

Draw the arms forward in front of the body, then back to start just under the water.

Teaching points
Back straight, arms and shoulders under the water, baby-bump tucked in, fingers together, and hands cupped.

Alternatives
Easy: Pump arms forward and back.

Ex 10.16 Squats

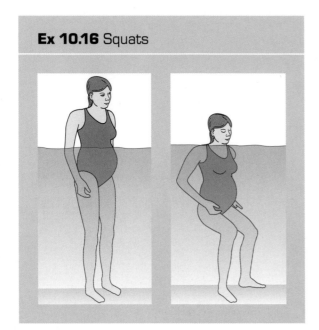

Ex 10.17 Pelvic tilts

Purpose

Knee and hip mobility.

Start position and instructions

- Standing in water at chest depth, with knees loose and joints not locked. Feet at least hip width apart (if comfortable).
- Bend at the knees and hips as if sitting into a chair, then raise up.

Teaching points

Hips, knees and toes all in line. Baby-bump facing forward. Heels down. Shoulders under the water.

Alternatives

- Easy: Shallower squats.
- Easy: Narrower stance for the feet.
- Harder: Deeper squats.

Purpose

Mobility for pelvis and education regarding pelvic and postural alignment.

Start position and instructions

Standing in water at chest depth, with knees loose and joints not locked and feet hip width apart or with one foot about one pace in front of the other. Whichever position the feet are in, weight should be evenly distributed through both legs. Gently tilt the pelvis backwards and forwards.

Teaching points

Shoulders under the water, hips and baby-bump bump facing forward. Heels down.

PREPARATORY STRETCHES

Ex 10.18 Gastrocnemius/calf stretch

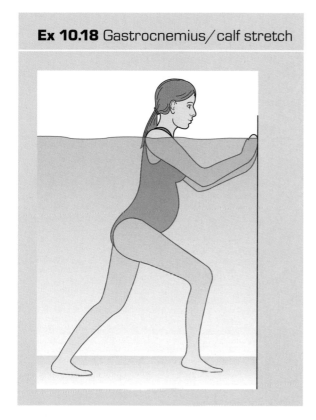

Ex 10.19 Hamstring stretch

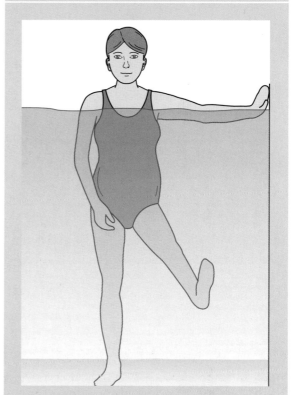

Start position and instructions

Stand facing the pool wall, with hands on the wall, shoulder width apart. One foot behind the other. Bend the front knee and lean forward keeping the back foot flat and stretching the back calf.

Teaching points

Shoulders under the water, baby-bump lifted and facing forwards. Hips forward, heels down. Weight should be evenly distributed through both legs.

Alternatives

Easy: Narrower stance.
Harder: Wider stance.

Start position and instructions

Standing side on to the pool wall, with hand on the wall for support. Lift one leg straight up in front. Knee joint soft on the standing leg.

Teaching points

Hips, knees and toes all in line. Keep heels down on the standing leg and shoulders under. Keep baby-bump lifted and hips level.

Alternatives

• Easy: Lower leg lift.
• Harder: Higher leg lift, but keep hips level.

Ex 10.20 Hip flexors stretch

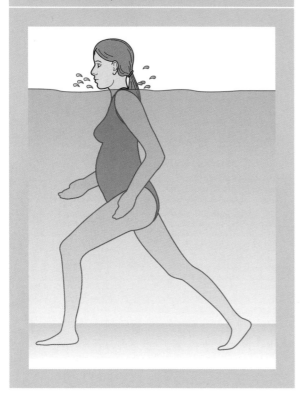

Ex 10.21 Adductors

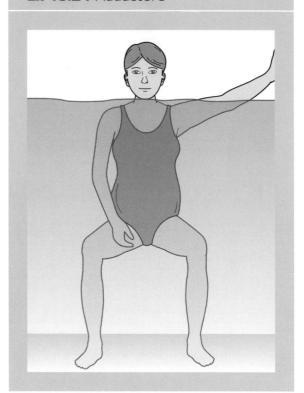

Start position and instructions

Standing side on to the pool wall, with hand on the wall for support. One foot behind the other. Weight should be evenly distributed through both legs. Bend knees and tuck pelvis under and lift baby-bump up and forwards.

Teaching points

Hips, knees and toes all in line. Keep shoulders under the water and the baby-bump lifted.

Alternatives

• Easy: Shallower knee bend.
• Harder: Deeper knee bend.

Start position and instructions

• Standing at chest depth, knees loose and joints not locked. Feet at least shoulder width apart.
• Bend the knees outwards and lower the body down so you feel a stretch in the inner thigh.

Teaching points

Shoulders under the water, brace abdominals, baby-bump lifted. Hips forward, heels down. Knees and toes in line.

Alternatives

• Easy: Narrower stance.
• Harder: Wider stance. Care to avoid any discomfort in the pelvis.

Ex 10.22 Pectorals/chest

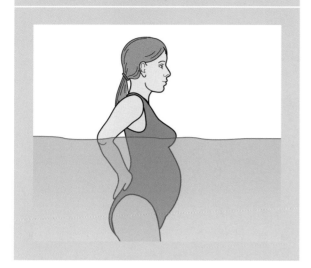

Ex 10.23 Triceps

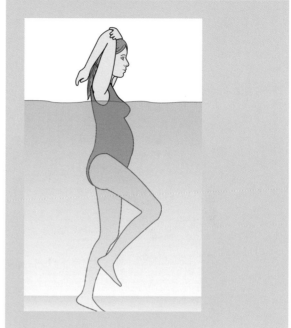

Purpose

Use the 'breaststroke arms' for a dynamic stretch to keep participants warm. Encourage full range of movement for effect – keeping the fingers closed with cupped hands will slow it right down.

Start position and instructions

Stand in water at chest depth, with knees loose and joints not locked and feet hip width apart or with one foot about one pace in front of the other. Weight should be evenly distributed through both legs. Hands behind body resting in small of back with fingertips pointing downwards.

Teaching points

Shoulders under the water, brace abdominals. Hips forward, heels down. Fingers together.

Alternatives

- Easy: Slice flat hands through the water.
- Easy: Open the fingers.
- Harder: Cup hands.

Start position and instructions

- Perform this whilst jogging/walking to maintain warmth.
- Standing in water at chest depth, with knees loose and joints not locked, and feet hip width apart or with one foot about one pace in front of the other. Whichever position the feet are in, weight should be evenly distributed through both legs. One hand over the shoulder, other arm supporting it at the elbow.

Teaching points

Shoulders under the water, abdominals in, hips and baby-bump facing forward. Heels down. Keep head up.

Alternatives

Easy: Smaller range of movement.

MAIN ACTIVITY EXERCISES
CARDIOVASCULAR/AEROBIC EXERCISES

All the pulse raising activities can also be used as cardiovascular exercises; the moves need to be bigger with a fuller range of movement and if participants are comfortable, they can add some more 'spring' to utilise the buoyancy of the water and increase the intensity of each exercise.

Additional exercises suitable for the cardiovascular section are listed below:

Ex 10.24 Jacks

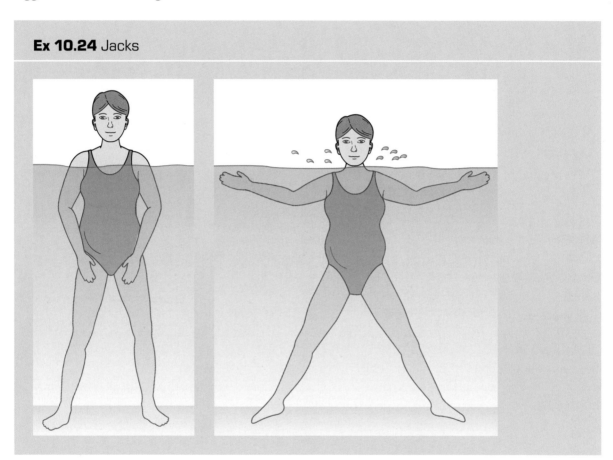

Purpose
Aerobic

Start position and instructions
Standing in water at chest depth, with knees loose and joints not locked. Spring up and take legs out to the sides, landing with feet apart.

Teaching points
Shoulders under the water, baby-bump lifted. Knees in line with toes, heels down on landing.

Alternatives
* Easy: Squats.
* Harder: More spring.

Ex 10.25 Aqua jog

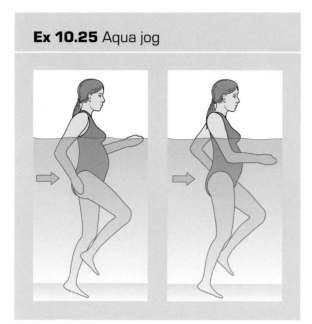

Ex 10. 26 Shuffles

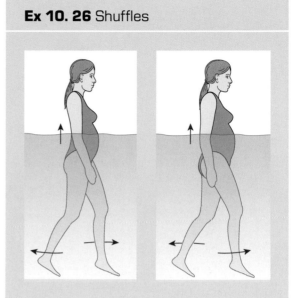

Purpose
Aerobic

Start position and instructions
Standing in water at chest depth, with knees loose and joints not locked. Lift legs into a march or jog and travel, pump arms in a running action.

Teaching points
Shoulders under the water, hips and baby-bump facing forward. Heels down.

Alternatives
Easy: Walk or lower jog.
Harder: More spring/faster jog.

Purpose
Aerobic

Start position and instructions
Standing in water at chest depth, with knees loose and joints not locked. Spring up and take one leg forward and one leg back. Repeat and change legs.

Teaching points
Shoulders under the water, brace abdominals and pull baby-bump in. Hips forward, heels down.

Alternatives
•   Easy: Less spring, keep legs narrower.
•   Harder: More spring, bigger movement.

Ex 10.27 Low kicks

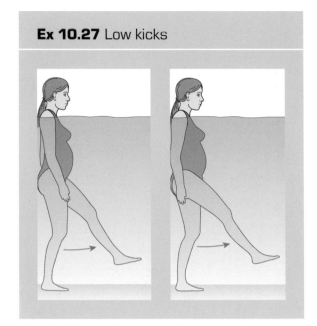

Purpose
Aerobic

Start position and instructions
Standing in water at chest depth, with knees loose and joints not locked. Lift leg straight in front of body then change legs.

Teaching points
Keep kicks low, knees bent. Abdominals and baby-bump tucked in. Heels down.

Alternatives
- Easy: Less spring, knee lifts.
- Harder: More spring.

Ex 10.28 Flutter kicks

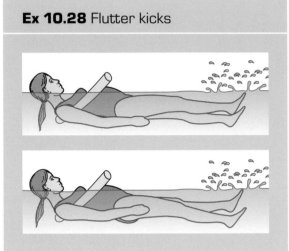

Purpose
To improve strength and endurance in the hip flexors and gluteals.

Start position and instructions
Floating on back with noodle under the shoulders for support. Keep legs together and straight at the knees. Kick legs up and down.

Teaching points
Try and lie back in the water with hips lifted towards the surface.

Alternatives
- This move could be performed lying on front with floats for support or holding onto pool wall.
- Just make sure that the head and neck stay in line with the rest of the back and there is no excessive arching.
- If floating on the back is difficult, try using a second noodle under the hips or lower back.
- Some may not wish to lie back due to lack of confidence or not wanting to get hair wet.

MUSCULAR STRENGTH AND ENDURANCE EXERCISES

Ex 10.29 Pool wall press-up and tricep dip

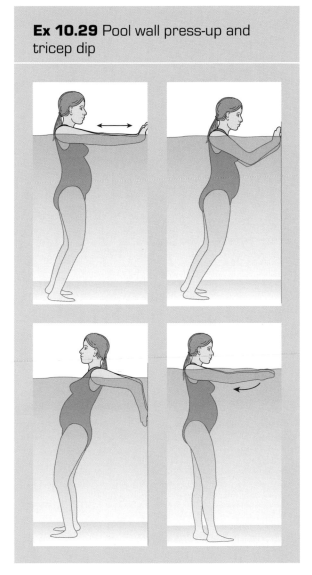

Purpose
To improve strength and endurance in the pectoral and triceps muscles.

Start position and instructions
Standing in water at chest depth, with knees loose and joints not locked. Hands on pool wall about shoulder width apart. Slowly lower chest towards wall by bending the elbows.

Teaching points
Keep elbows slightly bent as arms straighten. Keep the baby-bump lifted throughout the movement.

Alternatives
* Easy: Smaller movement.
* Harder: Triceps dips.

Ex 10.30 Breaststroke arm sweeps

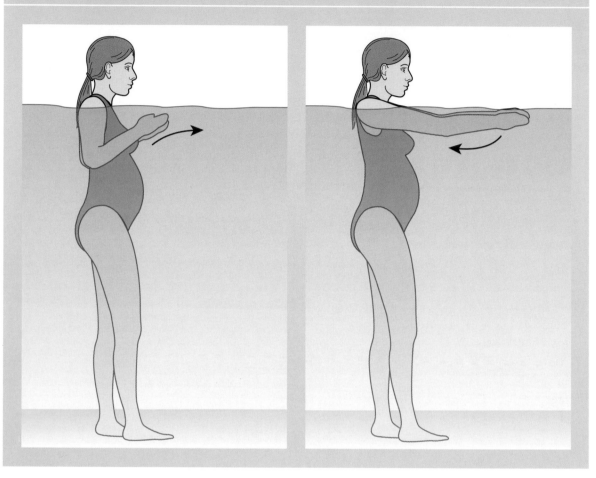

Purpose

To improve strength and endurance in the pectorals and trapezius muscles.

Start position and instructions

- Standing in water at chest depth, with knees loose and joints not locked, and feet hip width apart or with one foot about one pace in front of the other. Whichever position the feet are in, weight should be evenly distributed through both legs.

- Perform a breaststroke movement with the arms, keeping them under the water.

Teaching points

Shoulders under the water, brace abdominals. Hips forward, heels down. Fingers together.

Alternatives

- Easy: Fingers open or slicing the hands.
- Harder: Fingers closed, hands cupped, or wear aqua mitts, or hold float.

Ex 10.31 Biceps curl with mitts

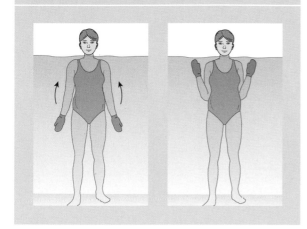

Ex 10.32 Seated balance (on noodle)

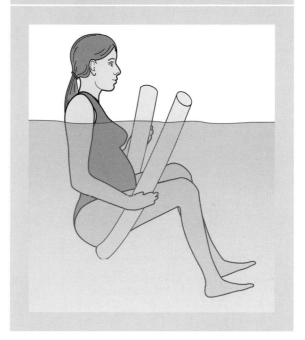

Purpose
To improve strength and endurance in the biceps.

Start position and instructions
*   Standing in water at chest depth, with knees loose and joints not locked, and feet hip width apart or with one foot about one pace in front of the other. Whichever position the feet are in, weight should be evenly distributed through both legs.
*   Keep the mitts palm up and sweep the hands up towards the shoulders, then return to starting position by the sides of the body.

Teaching points
Shoulders under the water, abdominals in, hips forward. Keep hands under the water throughout the movement.

Alternatives
*   Easy: Without dumbbell. Fingers open. Slicing hands.
*   Harder: Fingers together. Hands cupped. With float.

Purpose
To improve core strength and posture.

Start position and instructions
Sitting, balanced on a noodle shaped float with baby-bump pulled in and feet and knees together.

Teaching points
Keep back and neck long, ribcage lifted. Avoid holding the breath. Scull with hands for stability.

Alternatives
*   Easy: Use wall for added support.
*   Harder: Keep one hand still in lap.

Ex 10.33 Push and pull with noodle (with a partner)

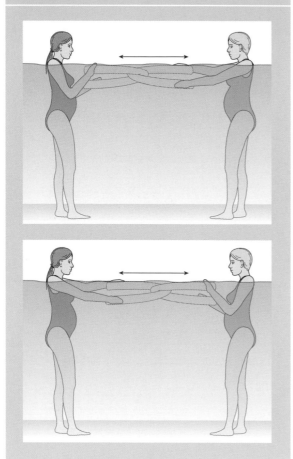

Purpose

To promote social interaction and fun. To improve strength and endurance in pectorals and trapezius.

Start position and instructions

Standing in water at chest depth, with knees loose and joints not locked with one foot about one pace in front of the other. Weight should be evenly distributed through both legs. Link floats with a partner and stand facing each other at arm's length. Pull the float towards you as partner resists the movement. Then partner tries to pull float as you resist the movement.

Teaching points

Shoulders under the water, brace abdominals. Hips forward, heels down. Try not to lock out elbows as arms are extended.

Alternatives

- Easy: Perform without a partner. Perform with a partner, but without a noodle and palms together.
- Harder: Increase resistance to the partner's movement.

Ex 10.34 Posture push

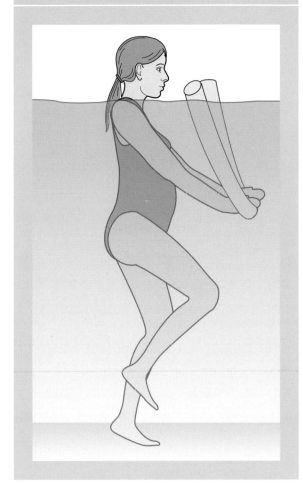

Purpose
To improve core strength and posture.

Start position and instructions
Standing in water at chest depth, with knees loose and joints not locked. Hold noodle in both hands about shoulder width apart. Push noodle down under the water to about hip level and extend arms forward. Walk forward pushing float in front like a supermarket trolley or buggy.

Teaching points
Shoulders under the water, brace abdominals. Hips forward, heels down.

Alternatives
- Easy: Perform without float with arms extended in front of body and palms forward.
- Harder: Increase speed.

COOLING DOWN
PULSE LOWERING
Any of the pulse raising exercises can be used to bring the intensity down during the cool down. Aim to gradually decrease the size of the 'spring' and possibly the speed of the movements in order to reduce heart rate and effort level.

COOL DOWN STRETCHES
Any of the preparatory stretches are suitable here, just hold them for a little longer to start to promote a feeling of well-being and relaxation. Remember that movement will still need to be included in between any static stretches to keep participants warm.

RELAXATION

Ex 10.35 Relaxation positions

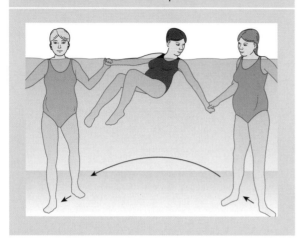

Start position and instructions

(a) Floating on back with noodle shaped float under the shoulders for support.

(b) Sitting, balanced on a noodle shaped float. Noodle under the thighs like sitting on a swing.

(c) Standing in water at chest depth, with knees loose and joints not locked. Participants in a circle holding hands. Start side-stepping round in a circle and every second person floats on their back.

Teaching points

(a): Keep legs together.

Notes

(a) and (b): These may not work if you have an odd number of participants. Some may not wish to lie back due to lack of confidence or not wanting to get hair wet.

OVERVIEW OF EXERCISES FOR AN AQUA-NATAL SESSION

Warm-up activities

- Walking/marching
- Breathing exercises
- Walking around pool
- Breaststroke arms
- Forward arm sweeps
- Pelvic floor contractions
- Knee lifts
- Leg curls
- Squats
- Preparatory stretches: calf, hamstrings, adductors, pectorals, triceps, hip flexors

Cardiovascular activities

- Side steps
- Jacks
- Aqua jog
- Shuffle
- Low forward kick

Muscular strength and endurance activities

- Wall press-up
- 'Pony' walking
- Seated balance (on float)
- Breaststroke arm sweeps
- Flutter kicks (at poolside or with float for support)
- Rear leg lifts
- Pram push-pram pull
- Posture push with float

Cool down/end of class activities

- Breathing exercises
- Pelvic floor contractions
- Cool down stretches: hamstrings, adductors, calf, pectorals, triceps, hip flexors

EXAMPLES OF TAI CHI STYLE MOVEMENTS

Figure 10.1 Single arm sweeps: arm sweeps across the body, hands scooping the water

Suitable for mobilising shoulders in the warm-up and cool down.

Figure 10.2 Double arm sweeps: arms sweep across the body, hands slicing the water

Suitable for mobilising shoulders and stretching pectorals and trapezius in the warm-up and cool down.

Figure 10.3 Downward arm sweeps: Arms sweep down in front of the body, palms down on downward phase, palms up on the way up

Suitable for mobilising shoulders and focusing breathing in the warm-up and cool down.

Figure 10.1 Single arm sweeps   **Figure 10.2** Double arm sweeps

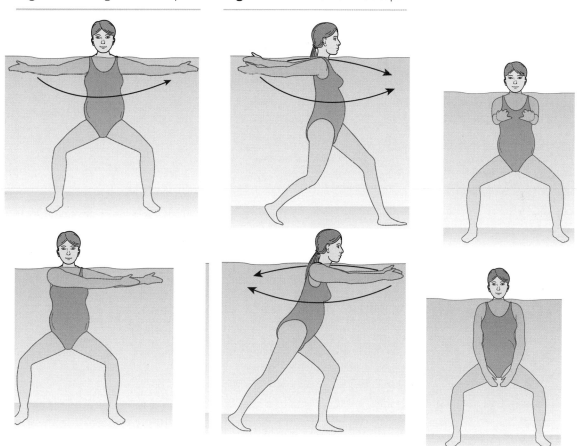

Figure 10.3 Downward arm sweeps

ADDITIONAL EXERCISES FOR THE POSTNATAL PERIOD

11

All the exercises listed in the prenatal section are appropriate for the postnatal period; however, there are further exercises that will help to regain pre-pregnancy fitness and shape. These can be included now the baby-bump has gone, centre of gravity returns to normal and abdominal muscles are re-aligned.

WARM-UP EXERCISES

See prenatal exercises in Chapter 10 for details.

MAIN ACTIVITY EXERCISES

Once the baby has been born and the woman has been cleared for a return to exercise, more vigorous activities can be included in the session. It is also appropriate to include specific exercises for the abdominal muscles, provided the 'rec check' is passed. Any of the exercises in Chapter 10 are also suitable.

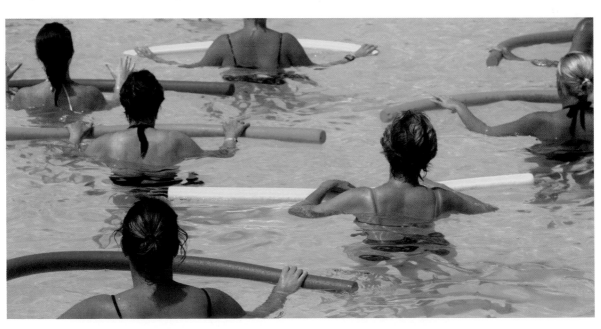

CARDIOVASCULAR EXERCISES

Ex 11.1 Rocking horse

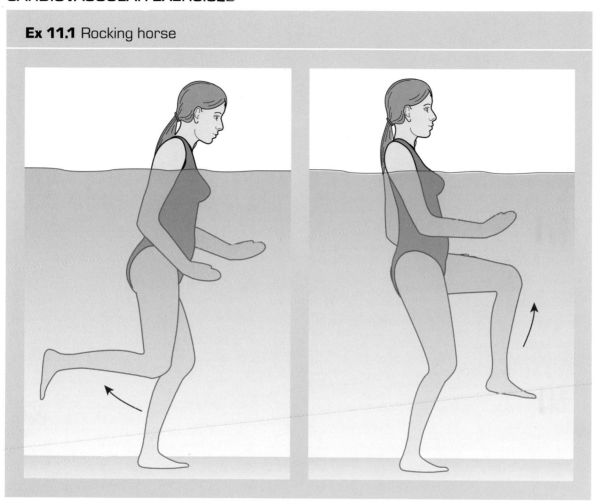

Purpose
Aerobic

Start position and instructions
Standing in water at chest depth, with knees loose and joints not locked with one foot about one pace in front of the other. Weight should be evenly distributed through both legs. Lift knee up on one leg, then swap legs and lift heel up to bottom on the other leg. Remember to swap leading leg after desired number of repetitions.

Teaching points
Abdominals tucked in. Heels down, knees soft on landing.

Alternatives
- Easy: Knee lifts.
- Harder: More spring.

Ex 11.2 Vertical jump

Ex 11.3 Tuck jump

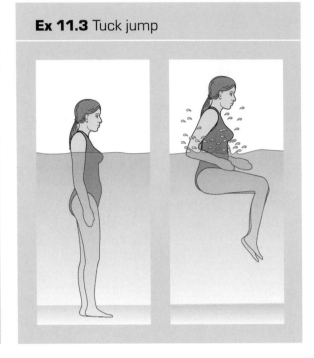

Purpose
Aerobic

Start position and instructions
Standing in water at chest depth, with knees loose
and joints not locked. Keeping legs together, jump
straight upwards out of the water.

Teaching points
Knees bent and heels down on landing.

Alternatives
Easy: Jog on the spot.
Harder: Higher jump, and circle arms up and out
of the water as you jump.

Purpose
Aerobic

Start position and instructions
Standing in water at chest depth, with knees loose
and joints not locked. Keep legs together, then
jump upwards, bringing both knees up towards
hips.

Teaching points
Knees bent and heels down on landing.

Alternatives
• Easy: Vertical jump. Less spring.
• Harder: Higher jump. Bring knees up higher.

Ex 11.4 Leap frog

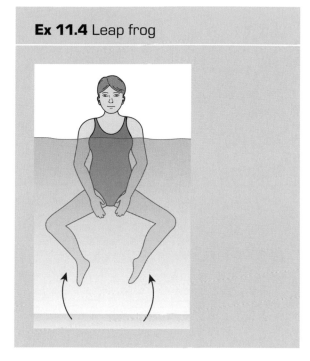

Purpose
Aerobic

Start position and instructions
Standing in water at chest depth, with knees loose and joints not locked. Jump up, taking knees up and out to the sides of the body.

Teaching points
Knees bent and heels down on landing.

Alternatives
*   Easy: Tuck jump or vertical jump. Less spring.
*   Harder: Higher jump. Lift knees up and out higher.

Ex 11.5 Gallops

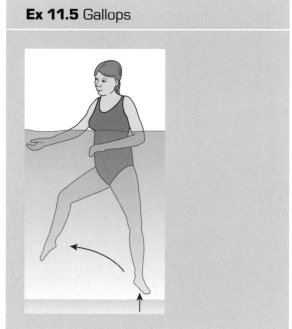

Purpose
Aerobic

Start position and instructions
Standing in water at chest depth, with knees loose and joints not locked. Facing forwards, take side steps with a spring.

Teaching points
Shoulders under the water, brace abdominals. Hips forward, heels down. Arms pull across body opposite to direction of travel. Fingers together, hands cupped.

Alternatives
*   Easy: Side steps.
*   Easy: Turn and walk in the direction of the side steps.
*   Harder: Higher spring. Wider step (care to avoid pelvic discomfort).

Ex 11.6 Power knee raise

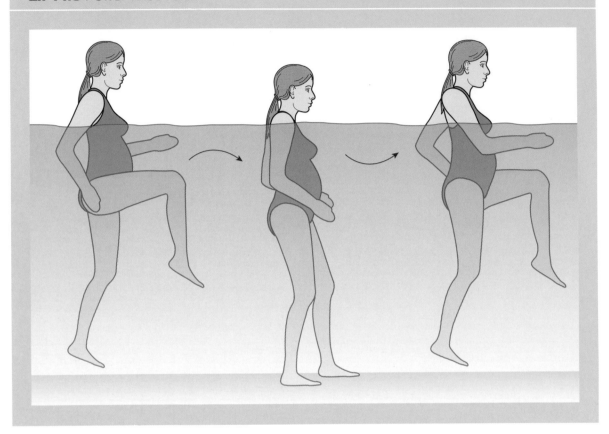

Purpose
Aerobic

Start position and instructions
Standing in water at chest depth, with knees loose and joints not locked. Jump and lift right knee, then switch legs and land back on right leg. Repeat starting left.

Teaching points
Hips, knees and toes all in line. Keep heels down and shoulders under the water.

Alternatives
- Easy: Knee lift.
- Harder: Higher knee lift and more spring.

Ex 11.7 Lateral raise with dumbbell floats

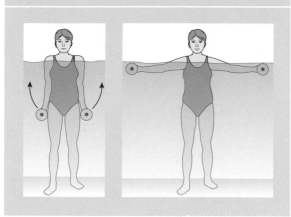

Ex 11.8 Leg extension with float

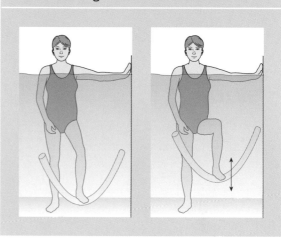

Purpose

To improve strength and endurance in latissimus dorsi.

Start position and instructions

Standing in water at chest depth, with knees loose and joints not locked, feet about hip width apart or with one foot about one pace in front of the other. Whichever position the feet are in, weight should be evenly distributed through both legs. Start with dumbbell float in each hand by side of body and slowly, with control, take them up to just under the surface of the water and then pull them slowly back under the water.

Teaching points

Shoulders under the water, abdominals in, hips forward.

Alternatives

*   Easy: No dumbbell floats in hands.
*   Harder: Speed up the movement, but maintain full range of movement.

Purpose

To improve strength and endurance in quadriceps and gluteals.

Start position and instructions

Standing in water at chest depth, with knees loose and joints not locked. One hand on pool wall for balance and stability. Stand on the noodle with one foot and raise knee up and down.

Teaching points

*   Keep heels down and shoulders under the water.
*   Keep abdominals pulled in. Try to keep hips level.

Alternatives

*   Easy: Smaller float under foot. Noodle under the thigh.
*   Harder: Without the wall for support.

ABDOMINAL EXERCISES

Ex 11.9 Abdominal pull in

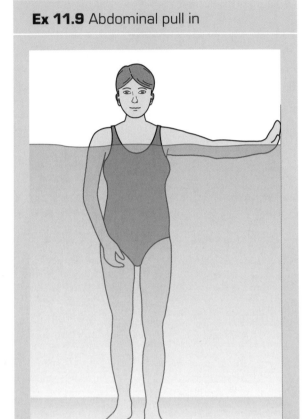

Purpose
To improve core strength and endurance.

Start position and instructions
- Standing in water at chest depth, with knees loose and joints not locked, feet about hip width apart or with one foot about one pace in front of the other. Whichever position the feet are in, weight should be evenly distributed through both legs.
- Focus on pulling in the abdominal muscles from belly button to pelvis; hold then release.

Teaching points
Brace abdominals. Avoid holding breath or gripping with buttocks.

Alternatives
- Easy: Have one hand on pool wall for added stability and balance.
- Harder: Perform this exercise whilst sitting on a noodle.
- Harder: Perform this exercise floating without support, in a sitting position.

Ex 11.10 Abdominal leg sweep

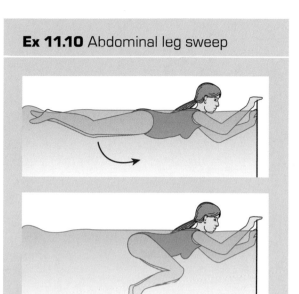

Ex 11.11 Triceps push down with noodle

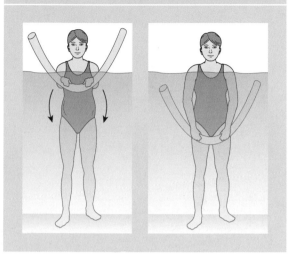

Purpose

To improve core strength and endurance.

Start position and instructions

Holding pool wall with both hands about shoulder width apart. Float horizontally on front with legs out straight behind body and feet and knees together. Sweep legs in towards body in a smooth, continuous movement.

Teaching points

Brace abdominals. Keep feet and knees together. Keep head looking forward to avoid arching the neck and spine.

Alternatives

* Easy: Standing abdominal pull in.
* Harder: Perform this exercise floating in the pool with a noodle in the hands instead of holding onto the pool wall.

Purpose

To improve strength and endurance in the triceps.

Start position and instructions

Standing in water at chest depth, with knees loose and joints not locked with one foot about one pace in front of the other. Weight should be evenly distributed through both legs. Hold noodle with the hands about shoulder width apart and then straighten arms to push the float under water.

Teaching points

Shoulders under the water, abdominals in, hips forward. Keep hands under the water throughout the movement.

Alternatives

* Easy: Without float. Fingers open.
* Harder: Perform this exercise with jogging or jacks or shuffles to challenge coordination and also maintain warmth.

Ex 11.12 Bent leg twists

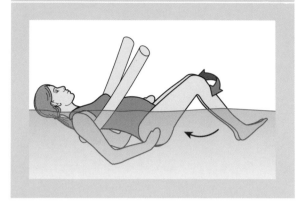

Purpose

To improve strength and endurance in the obliques.

Start position and instructions

Float horizontally on back. Noodle under shoulders and legs bent at the knees and feet together. Twist knees from side to side in a smooth, controlled movement.

Teaching points

Brace abdominals. Keep feet and knees together. Try to keep upper body still.

Alternatives

- Easy: Use wall for support.
- Harder: Try to float and perform the exercise without a noodle.
- If floating on the back is difficult, try using a second noodle under the hips or lower back.

Ex 11.13 Back to front leg sweeps

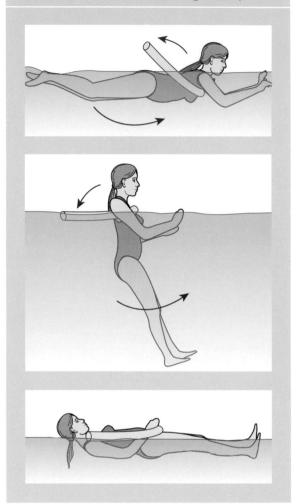

Purpose

To improve strength and endurance in the abdominals and core.

Start position and instructions

Float horizontally on front with noodle under arms and legs out straight behind body. Feet and knees together. Sweep legs forwards and under body in one smooth continuous move until they are all the way forwards and you are now floating on your back. Repeat leg sweeps to return to lying on front.

Teaching points

Brace abdominals. Keep feet and knees together.

Alternatives

*   Easy: Leg sweep at pool wall.
*   Harder: Try without the noodle.

Ex 11.14 Treading water

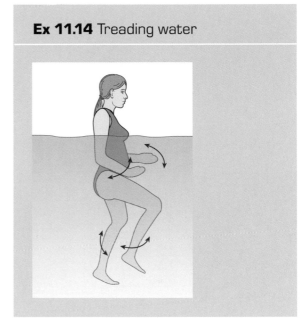

Purpose

To improve strength and endurance in the deep abdominal muscles.

Start position and instructions

Stand with feet about hip width apart or with one foot about one pace in front of the other. Start jogging and then lift knees off the pool floor so that the jogging continues in a floating position. Scull/circle the hands to aid stability and maintain buoyancy.

Teaching points

Brace abdominals. Keep back long and ribcage lifted. Avoid holding breath.

Alternatives

*   Easy: Use pool wall for added stability and balance.
*   Harder: Try sculling/circling with just one hand and raise the other hand out of the water.

COMBINATION POSTNATAL ABDOMINAL EXERCISES IN THE POOL

Adapted from: *Lumbar Stabilization, Why and How?* Beth Scalone, PT, DPT, OCS.

Level 1

Ex 11.15 Chest-deep water walking

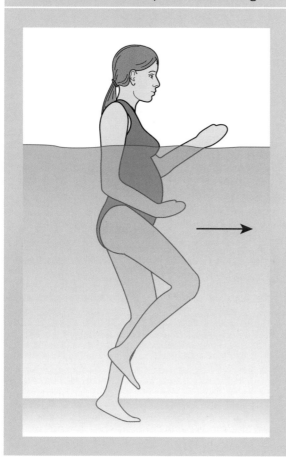

Purpose
To improve stamina and endurance and posture.

Start position and instructions
Chest deep in the pool. Posture upright and abdominals pulled in. Walk forwards.

Teaching points
Maintain neutral spine and add upper limb movement, slow and medium speeds. Keep abdominals pulled in.

Alternatives
*   Easy: Shallower water. Start leaning against the side of the pool then progress to mid-pool without support.
*   Harder: Add higher knee lifting and increase speed. Add resistance by pushing a noodle forward in front of the body (see Posture push exercise, p 98).

Ex 11.16 Chest-deep water walking forwards, backwards and side stepping

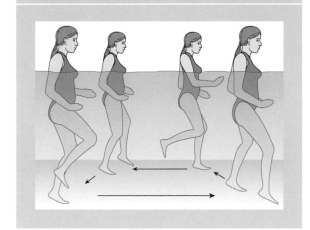

Purpose

To improve cardiovascular fitness and improve endurance in the legs.

Start position and instructions

Chest deep in the pool. Posture upright and abdominals pulled in. Walk forwards, sideways, backwards and sideways in a square formation.

Teaching points

Maintain neutral spine and add upper limb movement. Keep abdominals pulled in.

Alternatives

Easy: Shallower water. Start leaning against pool side then progress to mid-pool without support. Harder: Faster movements.

Level 2 Basic

Ex 11.17 Scissor legs

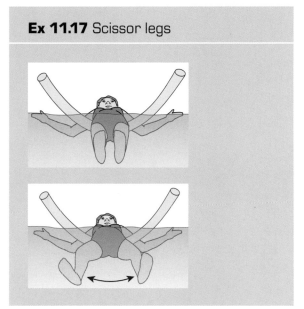

Purpose

To improve strength of the abductor and adductor muscles.

Start position and instructions

Floating on back with noodle under the shoulders for support. Keep legs together and straight at the knees, then slowly push legs out to the sides and back together again.

Teaching points

Try to lie back in the water with hips lifted towards the surface.

Alternatives

*   Easy: Smaller movements.
*   Harder: Bigger or faster movements. Try without noodle for support.
*   If floating on the back is difficult, try using a second noodle under the hips or lower back.

Ex 11.18 Forward and backward bicycle

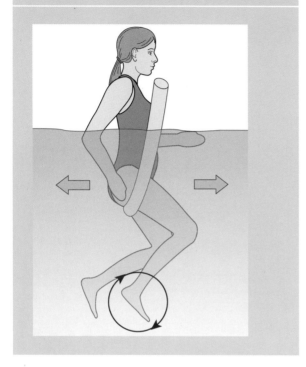

Purpose
To improve cardiovascular fitness.

Start position and instructions
Sitting balanced on a noodle shaped float with abdominals pulled in. Start with feet and knees together, then cycle the legs to travel off the spot.

Teaching points
Keep back and neck long, ribcage lifted. Avoid holding the breath. Scull with hands for stability.

Alternatives
- Easy: Use pool wall for support.
- Harder: Try sculling with just one hand and raising the other one out of the water.

Level 3 Intermediate

Ex 11.19 Sitting on the float with arm exercises

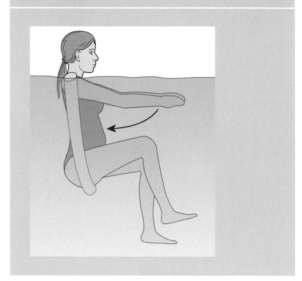

Purpose
To improve strength and endurance in the arm muscles.

Start position and instructions
Sitting balanced on a noodle shaped float with abs pulled in and feet and knees together. Perform arm exercises such as breaststroke arms, biceps curls.

Teaching points
Keep back and neck long, ribcage lifted. Avoid breath holding.

Alternatives
- Easy: Scull with hands instead of arm exercises OR use pool wall for support with one arm and perform the arm exercise on one arm at a time.
- Harder: Increase speed or range of arm movement.

Ex 11.20 L-sit float and row

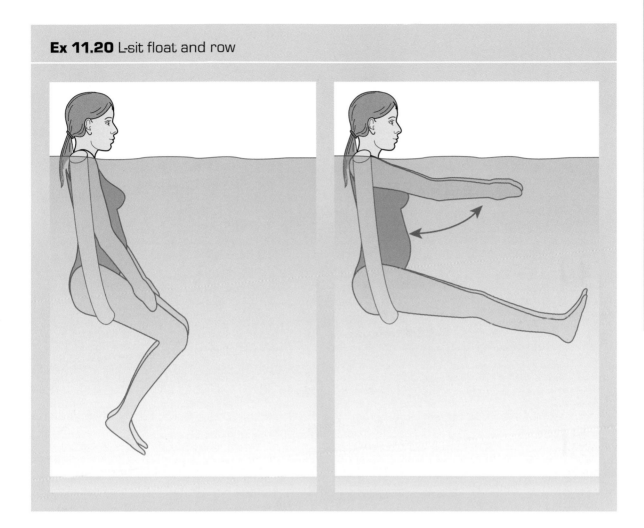

Purpose

To improve stamina in the arms.

Start position and instructions

Sitting balanced on a noodle, abs pulled in and feet and knees together. Slowly straighten legs straight out in front. Row arms back and forward.

Teaching points

Keep back and neck long, ribcage lifted. Avoid holding the breath.

Alternatives

- Easy: Scull with hands for stability instead of rowing.
- Harder: Increase speed.

Ex 11.21 L-sit float with breaststroke legs

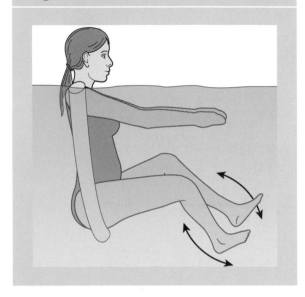

Purpose
To improve endurance in the abdominal, hip and leg muscles.

Start position and instructions
Floating on back with noodle under the shoulders for support. Keep legs together and straight at the knees, then slowly move legs out to the side in a breaststroke leg action.

Teaching points
Try and lie back in the water with hips lifted towards the surface.

Alternatives
- Easy: Smaller movements.
- Harder: Bigger or faster movements. Try without noodle for support. If floating on the back is difficult, try using a second noodle under the hips or lower back.

Level 4 Advanced

Ex 11.22 'Skipping' with float

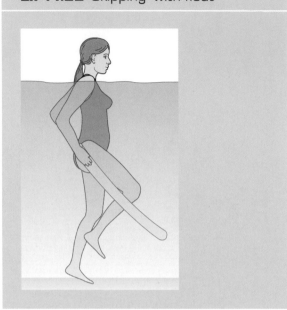

Purpose
To improve cardiovascular fitness.

Start position and instructions
Stand with feet about hip width apart or with one foot about one pace in front of the other. Hold one end of noodle in each hand and use it like a skipping rope, jumping over it one foot at a time.

Teaching points
Brace abdominals. Keep back long and ribcage lifted. Avoid holding breath.

Alternatives
- Easy: Try without noodle and use 'imaginary' skipping rope.
- Harder: Jump over the noodle with two feet at a time.

Ex 11.23 Side tucks

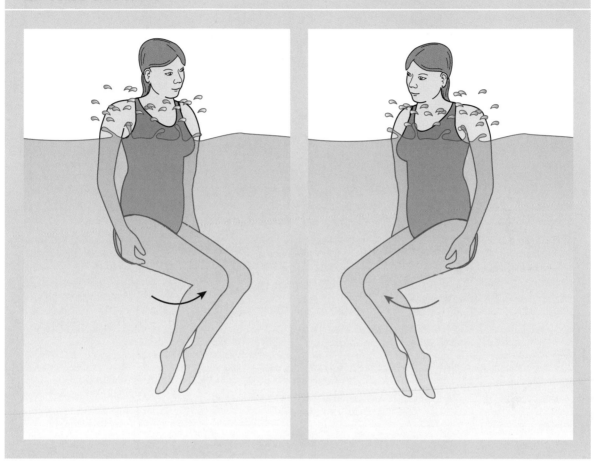

Purpose

To improve cardiovascular fitness.

Start position and instructions

Standing in water at chest depth, with knees loose and joints not locked. Keep legs together, then jump upwards and twist lower body, bringing both knees up towards one side, then repeat to jump and twist to the other side.

Teaching points

Knees bent and heels down on landing.

Alternatives

- Easy: Tuck jump. Less spring.
- Harder: Higher jump. Bring knees up higher.

Ex 11.24 Leg sweeps through front to back, side to side

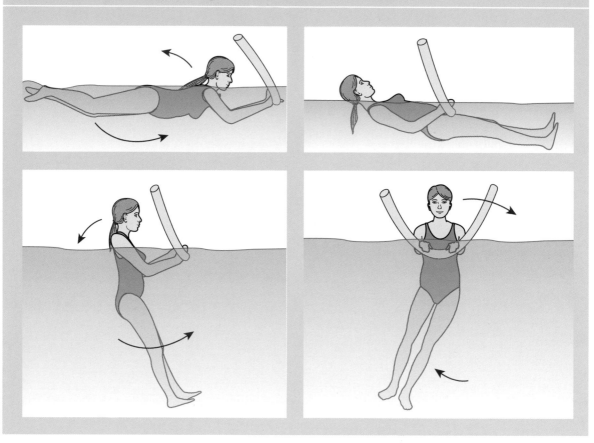

Purpose
To strengthen the abdominal muscles.

Start position and instructions
Float horizontally on front with noodle in hands and legs out straight behind body. Feet and knees together. Sweep legs forwards and under body in one smooth continuous move until they are all the way forwards and you are now floating on your back. Then sweep legs under body from one side to the other before returning to the start position lying on front.

Teaching points
Brace abdominals. Keep feet and knees together.

Alternatives
- Easy: Forward and back leg sweeps only.
- Harder: Without the support of a noodle.

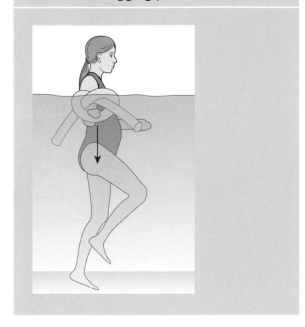

Ex 11.25 Jogging push downs

Purpose

To improve stamina and endurance.

Start position and instructions

Standing in water at chest depth, with knees loose and joints not locked. Noodle tied in a knot in one hand. Start to jog, then lean to the side and straighten the arm to push noodle under the water. Repeat for desired repetitions then swap sides.

Teaching points

Knees bent and heels down on landing. Try to keep elbow loose and not locked as it is straightened.

Alternatives

• Easy: No noodle in hand.
• Harder: Try performing this with a leg curl exercise instead of the jog. Add more spring.

COOLING DOWN
PULSE LOWERING

The aim of the cool down section is to return the heart and breathing rates back to a steady pre-exercise state. This is achieved by reducing the intensity and impact or by reversing the moves from the pulse raising section. Again, due to the water properties, this section can be a little quicker than on land, approximately 3–4 minutes, but it still needs to be smooth and very gradual. Take time to chat to your participants so you can tell from their breathing that they are getting back to a comfortable state. Breathing may still be a bit heavier than normal, but individuals should be able to talk freely. Most importantly, they should still feel warm.

POST-WORKOUT STRETCHES

All muscles worked in the session should be stretched during the cool down. However, prolonged (developmental) stretching, aimed at improving flexibility, is not appropriate until around five months post delivery, due to the continued effects of relaxin on the joints and the risk of stretching ligaments and tendons. Participants could also get very cold and uncomfortable during this time. Shorter hold stretches, aimed at maintaining flexibility, incorporating some movement in between as in the warm-up, are the best way to go. These static stretches can be done using the pool wall, the lane marker or a float for support. Offer alternatives for the more or less flexible participants and check too that individuals are not getting cold.

Finish with a short relaxation exercise to promote well-being.

Any of the exercises from the prenatal section can be used in the cool down.

Overall this final section of the class should take about 5–6 minutes. Including a little bit of relaxation here may offer some welcome 'me-time' for any participant feeling tired and stressed with the efforts of looking after a new baby.

OVERVIEW OF EXERCISES FOR A POSTNATAL AQUA SESSION

Warm-up activities

- Walking/marching
- Breaststroke arms
- Forward arm sweeps
- Pelvic floor contractions
- Knee lifts
- Leg curls
- Squats
- Prep stretches: hamstrings, calf, adductors, pectorals, triceps, hip flexors

Cardiovascular activities

- Side steps
- Jacks
- Aqua jog
- Shuffle
- Forward kick
- Rocking horse
- Vertical jump
- Tuck jump
- Leap frog
- Gallops
- Power knee raise

Muscular strength and endurance activities

- Triceps pushdown and float
- Lateral raise with floats
- Pectoral flye with float
- Leg extension with float

Abdominal exercises

- Abdominal pull in
- Abdominal leg sweep
- Bent leg twists
- Back to front leg sweeps
- Treading water
- L-sit float and row arms

Cool down/end of class activities

- Pelvic floor contractions
- Stretches: calf, hamstrings, hip flexors, adductors, pectorals, triceps

SAMPLE CLASSES

12

We have provided samples of warm-ups, main activities and cool downs that can be mixed and matched to provide a range of classes to suit all abilities and provide variety for your sessions. All the exercises are included in chapters 10 and 11 and alternatives are provided to enable you to include a range of fitness levels in your sessions.

PRENATAL WARM-UPS
WARM-UP 1

Table 12.1	Prenatal warm-up 1		
Exercises	**Purpose**	**Teaching points**	**Alternatives** **Easier (E) or harder (H)**
PULSE RAISING/MOBILITY			
Posture check			
Jogging in large circle around the pool	Pulse raising/ warming	• Shoulders underwater • Hips level and facing forward • Baby-bump lifted • Place heels down	• E: March on the spot • H: High knees jog • Slower participants jog on the inside, faster participants on outside of the circle
Single arm sweeps across body (Tai chi style, see p. 101)	Mobilising shoulders	• Shoulders underwater • Abdominals pulled in	• E: Smaller range of movement • H: Larger range of movement

Table 12.1	Prenatal warm-up 1 (cont.)		
Shallow squats*	Mobilising knees and hips, pulse raising	• Shoulders underwater • Hips, knees and toes all in line • Baby-bump lifted and facing forward • Heels down	• E: Shallower squats • E: Narrower stance for the feet • H: Deeper squats
Arm sweeps forward and back (Tai chi style)	Mobilising shoulders	• Shoulders underwater • Abdominals pulled in	• E: Smaller range of movement • H: Larger range of movement
Side steps R x 4 Squat on the spot x 4 Repeat to L	Mobilising hips and knees/pulse raising	• Shoulders underwater • Hips, knees and toes all in line • Baby-bump lifted and facing forward • Heels down	• E: Smaller side steps • E: Shallower squats • H: Faster side steps • H: Deeper squats
Knee lifts	Mobilising hips and knees/pulse raising	• Hips, knees and toes all in line • Keep heels down and shoulders underwater	• E: Smaller lifts • H: Bigger moves • H: Add a spring • If the baby-bump is large, reduce height of knee lift or take knee slightly out to the side
Repeat from * x 2	Pulse raising	See above	• H: Faster or larger moves
STRETCHES			
Hamstring stretch	Static stretch for hamstrings	• Hips, knees and toes all in line • Keep heels down on the standing leg and shoulders under • Keep baby-bump lifted and hips level	• E: Lower leg lift • H: Higher leg lift, but keep hips level
Calf stretch	Static stretch for calf	• Shoulders underwater, baby-bump lifted and facing forwards • Hips forward, heels down • Weight should be evenly distributed through both legs	

Table 12.1	Prenatal warm-up 1 (cont.)		
Breaststroke arms	Dynamic stretch for pectorals	• Shoulders underwater, brace abdominals • Hips forward, heels down • Fingers together	• E: Slice hands through the water with a flat hand • Open the fingers
Jog on the spot and stretch triceps	Triceps stretch (moving to keep warm)	• Shoulders underwater, abdominals in • Hips and baby-bump facing forward • Avoid arching the back • Keep head up	• E: Elbow lower • H: Raise elbow higher to increase range of stretch
Squats	Mobility and to keep warm	See above	See above
REWARM			
Side steps R**	CV/aerobic		
Squats	See above	See above	See above
Repeat all L			
Jog forward	CV/aerobic	• Shoulders underwater, hips and baby-bump facing forward • Heels down	• E: Stay on the spot and jog/march • H: Lift knees higher, travel further
Low leg kicks on the spot	CV/aerobic	• Keep kicks low, knees bent • Abdominals and baby-bump pulled in • Heels down	• E: Less spring • E: Knee lifts • H: More spring
Jog back/leg kick on the spot	CV/aerobic	• Shoulders underwater, hips and baby-bump facing forward • Heels down	• E: Stay on the spot and jog/march • H: Lift knees higher, travel further
Repeat twice from **	Aim to increase range of movement slightly to increase intensity		

WARM-UP 2

Table 12.2	Prenatal warm-up 2		
Exercises	**Purpose**	**Teaching points**	**Alternatives**
Posture check			
Jogging in large circle around the pool	Pulse raising/ warming	• Shoulders underwater • Hips level and facing forward • Baby-bump lifted • Place heels down	• E: March on the spot • H: High knees jog • Slower participants jog on the inside, faster participants on outside of the circle
Breaststroke arms	Dynamic stretch for pectorals	• Shoulders underwater, brace abdominals • Hips forward, heels down • Fingers together	• E: Slice hands through the water with a flat hand • E: Open the fingers
Leg curls*	Pulse raising and knee mobility	• Keep heels down and shoulders underwater • Keep baby-bump pulled in and hips facing forward	• E: Smaller curl • E: Jog • H: Add a spring as legs change
Downward arm sweeps (Tai chi style, see p. 101)	Mobilising shoulders	• Shoulders underwater • Abdominals pulled in	• E: Smaller range of movement • H: Larger range of movement
Side steps R and low kick on the spot	Mobilising knees and hips, pulse raising	• Shoulders underwater • Hips, knees and toes all in line • Baby-bump lifted and facing forward • Heels down	• E: Smaller side steps • E: Less spring on kicks • E: Knee lifts • H: Wider side steps • H: More spring on kicks
Repeat to the left			
Jacks	Mobilising hips and knees/pulse raising	• Shoulders underwater • Hips, knees and toes all in line • Baby-bump lifted and facing forward • Heels down	• E: Squats • H: More spring

Table 12.2   Prenatal warm-up 2 (cont.)

Repeat twice from *			
Arm sweeps forward and back (Tai chi style, see p. 101)	Mobilising shoulders	• Shoulders underwater • Abdominals pulled in	• E: Smaller range of movement • H: Larger range of movement
Side steps R x 4 Squat on the spot x 4 Repeat to L	Mobilising hips and knees/pulse raising	• Shoulders underwater • Hips, knees and toes all in line • Baby-bump lifted and facing forward • Heels down	• E: Smaller side steps • E: Shallower squats • H: Faster side steps • H: Deeper squats
Knee lifts	Mobilising hips and knees/pulse raising	• Hips, knees and toes all in line • Keep heels down and shoulders underwater	• E: Smaller lifts • H: Bigger moves • H: Add a spring • If baby-bump is large, reduce height of knee lift or take knee slightly out to the side
Repeat from * x 2	Pulse raising	See above	• H: Faster or larger moves

STRETCHES

Hamstring stretch	Static stretch for hamstrings	• Hips, knees and toes all in line • Keep heels down on the standing leg and shoulders underwater • Keep baby-bump lifted and hips level	• E: Lower leg lift • H: Higher leg lift, but keep hips level
Calf stretch	Static stretch for calf	• Shoulders underwater, baby-bump lifted and facing forward • Hips forward, heels down • Weight should be evenly distributed through both legs	• E: Narrower stance • H: Wider stance

Table 12.2	Prenatal warm-up 2 (cont.)		
Jog on the spot and stretch triceps	Triceps stretch (moving to keep warm)	• Shoulders underwater, abdominals in, hips and baby-bump facing forward • Heels down • Keep head up	• E: Elbow lower • H: Greater range of stretch
Pectoral stretch/ Breaststroke arms	Dynamic stretch for pectorals	• Shoulders underwater, brace abdominals • Hips forward, heels down • Fingers together	• E: Slice hands through the water with a flat hand • E: Open the fingers • H: Cup hands
Side steps R and jacks	Pulse raising	See above	See above
Hip flexor stretch	Static stretch for the hip flexors	• Shoulders underwater, brace abdominals, baby-bump lifted • Hips forward, front heel down, back heel lifted • Knees and toes in line	• E: Shallower knee bend • H: Deeper knee bend • Avoid any discomfort in the pelvis
Side steps L and jacks	Pulse raising	See above	See above
REWARM			
Side steps right**	See above	See above	See above
Shuffle	CV/aerobic	• Shoulders underwater, brace abdominals and pull baby-bump in • Hips forward, heels down	• E: Less spring, keep legs narrower • H: More spring, bigger movement
Repeat all L			
Fast jog on the spot	CV/aerobic	• Shoulders underwater, hips and baby-bump facing forward • Heels down	• E: Slower jog or march • H: Lift knees higher

Table 12.2	Prenatal warm-up 2 (cont.)		
Knee lifts on the spot	CV/aerobic	• Hips, knees and toes all in line • Keep heels down and shoulders underwater	• E: Smaller moves • H: Bigger moves • H: Add a spring • If baby-bump is large, reduce height of knee lift or take knee slightly out to the side
Fast jog on the spot	CV/aerobic	• Shoulders underwater, hips and baby-bump facing forward • Heels down	• E: Slower jog or march • H: Lift knees higher
Repeat twice from **	Aim to increase range of movement slightly to increase intensity		

WARM-UP 3

Table 12.3	Prenatal warm-up 3		
Exercises	**Purpose**	**Teaching points**	**Alternatives**
Posture check			
Jogging in large circle around the pool	Pulse raising/ warming	• Shoulders underwater • Hips level and facing forward • Baby-bump lifted • Place heels down	• E: March on the spot • H: High knees jog • Slower participants jog on the inside, faster participants on outside of the circle
Single arm sweeps across body (Tai chi style, see p. 101)	Mobilising shoulders	• Shoulders underwater • Abdominals pulled in	• E: Smaller range of movement • H: Larger range of movement

Table 12.3	Prenatal warm-up 3 (cont.)		
Shallow squats*	Mobilising knees and hips, pulse raising	• Shoulders underwater • Hips, knees and toes all in line • Baby-bump lifted and facing forward • Heels down	• E: Shallower squats • E: Narrower stance for the feet • H: Deeper squats
Downward arm sweeps (Tai chi style, see p. 101)	Mobilising shoulders	• Shoulders underwater • Abdominals pulled in	• E: Smaller range of movement • H: Larger range of movement
Jog forwards and shuffle on the spot	Mobilising knees, ankles and hips and pulse raising	• Shoulders underwater, hips and baby-bump facing forward • Heels down	• E: Stay on the spot and jog/march • H: Lift knees higher, travel further
Jog backwards and shuffle on the spot	Mobilising knees, ankles and hips and pulse raising	• Shoulders underwater, hips and baby-bump facing forward • Heels down	• E: Stay on the spot and jog/march • H: Lift knees higher, travel further

TURN 90°

Repeat jog and shuffle as above. Continue to turn and jog etc. until facing front again

Knee lifts	Mobilising hips and knees/pulse raising	• Hips, knees and toes all in line • Keep heels down and shoulders underwater	• E: Smaller lifts • H: Bigger moves • H: Add a spring • If baby-bump is large, reduce height of knee lift or take knee slightly out to the side
Hamstring stretch	Static stretch for hamstrings	• Hips, knees and toes all in line • Keep heels down on the standing leg and shoulders underwater • Keep baby-bump lifted and hips level	• E: Lower leg lift • H: Higher leg lift, but keep hips level
Calf stretch	Static stretch for calf	• Shoulders underwater, baby-bump lifted and facing forward • Hips forward, heels down • Weight should be evenly distributed through both legs	• E: Narrower stance • H: Wider stance

Table 12.3	Prenatal warm-up 3 (cont.)		
Jog on the spot and stretch triceps	Triceps stretch (moving to keep warm)	• Shoulders underwater, abdominals in, hips and baby-bump facing forward • Heels down • Keep head up	• E: Elbow lower • H: Greater range of stretch
Pectoral stretch/ Breaststroke arms	Dynamic stretch for pectorals	• Shoulders underwater, brace abdominals • Hips forward, heels down • Fingers together	• E: Slice hands through the water with a flat hand • E: Open the fingers • H: Cup hands
REWARM			
Squats	Mobility and to keep warm	See above	See above
Side steps R and low kick on the spot**	Mobilising knees and hips, pulse raising	• Shoulders underwater • Hips, knees and toes all in line • Baby-bump lifted and facing forward • Heels down	• E: Smaller side steps • E: Less spring on kicks • E: Knee lifts • H: Wider side steps • H: More spring on kicks
Repeat to the left			
Jog forwards Jacks on the spot	CV/aerobic	• Shoulders underwater, brace abdominals and pull baby-bump in • Hips forward, heels down	• E: Less spring, keep legs narrower • H: More spring, bigger movement
Jog backwards Jacks on the spot	CV/aerobic	• Shoulders underwater, brace abdominals and pull baby-bump in • Hips forward, heels down	• E: Less spring, keep legs narrower • H: More spring, bigger movement
Repeat twice from **	Aim to increase range of movement slightly to increase intensity		

WARM-UP 4

Table 12.4	Prenatal warm-up 4		
Exercises	**Purpose**	**Teaching points**	**Alternatives**
Posture check			
Jogging in large circle around the pool	Pulse raising/ warming	• Shoulders underwater • Hips level and facing forward • Baby-bump lifted • Place heels down	• E: March on the spot • H: High knees jog • Slower participants jog on the inside, faster participants on outside of the circle
Forward arm pushes	Mobilising shoulders and elbows	• Shoulders underwater • Abdominals pulled in	• E: Smaller range of movement • H: Larger range of movement
Low leg kicks*	Mobilising knees and hips, pulse raising	• Shoulders underwater • Hips, knees and toes all in line • Baby-bump lifted and facing forward • Heels down	• E: Shallower squats • E: Narrower stance for the feet • H: Deeper squats
Arm sweeps forward and back (Tai chi style, see p. 101)	Mobilising shoulders	• Shoulders underwater • Abdominals pulled in	• E: Smaller range of movement • H: Larger range of movement
Side steps R x 4 Squat on the spot x 4 Repeat to L	Mobilising hips and knees/pulse raising	• Shoulders underwater • Hips, knees and toes all in line • Baby-bump lifted and facing forward • Heels down	• E: Smaller side steps • E: Shallower squats • H: Faster side steps • H: Deeper squats
Shuffle	Pulse raising	• Shoulders underwater, brace abdominals and pull baby-bump in • Hips forward, heels down	• E: Less spring, keep legs narrower • H: More spring, bigger movement
Repeat twice from *			

Table 12.4	Prenatal warm-up 4 (cont.)		

STRETCHES

Hamstring stretch	Static stretch for hamstrings	• Hips, knees and toes all in line • Keep heels down on the standing leg and shoulders underwater • Keep baby-bump lifted and hips level	• E: Lower leg lift • H: Higher leg lift, but keep hips level
Calf stretch	Static stretch for calf	• Shoulders underwater, baby-bump lifted and facing forward • Hips forward, heels down • Weight should be evenly distributed through both legs	• E: Narrower stance • H: Wider stance
Jog on the spot and stretch triceps	Triceps stretch (moving to keep warm)	• Shoulders underwater, abdominals in, hips and baby-bump facing forward • Heels down • Keep head up	• E: Elbow lower • H: Greater range of stretch
Pectoral stretch/ Breaststroke arms	Dynamic stretch for pectorals	• Shoulders underwater, brace abdominals • Hips forward, heels down • Fingers together	• E: Slice hands through the water with a flat hand • E: Open the fingers • H: Cup hands
Squats	Mobility and to keep warm	See above	See above

REWARM

Side steps R and jog forwards**	Mobilising knees and hips, pulse raising	• Shoulders underwater • Hips, knees and toes all in line • Baby-bump lifted and facing forward • Heels down	• E: Smaller side steps • E: Knee lifts • E: March in place • H: Wider side steps • H: High knees on jog
Side steps L and jog backwards (this gives a square pattern)	Mobilising knees and hips, pulse raising	• Shoulders underwater • Hips, knees and toes all in line • Baby-bump lifted and facing forward • Heels down	• E: Smaller side steps • E: Knee lifts • E: March on the spot • H: Wider side steps • H: More high knees on jog

Table 12.4	Prenatal warm-up 4 (cont.)		
Knee lifts	CV/aerobic	• Hips, knees and toes all in line • Keep heels down and shoulders underwater	• E: Smaller moves • H: Bigger moves • H: Add a spring • If baby-bump is large, reduce height of knee lift or take knee slightly out to the side
Repeat twice from **	Aim to increase range of movement slightly to increase intensity		

AQUA EXERCISE

PRENATAL MAIN ACTIVITY WORKOUTS
PRENATAL MAIN ACTIVITY 1 – CARDIOVASCULAR CIRCUIT

Table 12.5	Prenatal main activity workout 1 – cardiovascular circuit		
Exercises	**Purpose**	**Teaching points**	**Alternatives**
Posture reinforcement			
Circuit station 1 Knee lifts	To improve cardiovascular/ aerobic fitness	• Hips, knees and toes all in line • Keep heels down and shoulders underwater	• E: Smaller moves • H: Bigger moves • H: Add a spring • If baby-bump is large, reduce height of knee lift or take knee slightly out to the side
Circuit station 2 Shuffles		• Shoulders underwater, brace abdominals and pull baby-bump in • Hips forward, heels down	• E: Less spring, keep legs narrower • H: More spring, bigger movement
Circuit station 3 Jacks		• Shoulders underwater, baby-bump lifted • Knees in line with toes, heels down on landing	• E: Squats • H: More spring
Circuit station 4 Leg curls		• Keep heels down and shoulders underwater • Keep baby-bump pulled in and hips facing forward	• E: Smaller curl • E: Jog • H: Add a spring as legs change
Circuit station 5 Low kicks forward		• Keep kicks low, knees bent • Abdominals and baby-bump tucked in • Heels down	• E: Less spring, knee lifts • H: More spring
Circuit station 6 Jogging		• Shoulders underwater, hips and baby-bump facing forward • Heels down	• Adjust the speed of the jog/ march, smaller march on the spot

PRENATAL MAIN ACTIVITY 2 – CHOREOGRAPHED ROUTINE

Table 12.6	Prenatal main activity workout 2 – choreographed routine		
Exercises	**Purpose**	**Teaching points**	**Alternatives**
Posture reinforcement			
Block 1 Side steps R x 4 Shuffle on the spot Side steps L x 4 Shuffle on the spot Repeat	To improve cardiovascular/ aerobic fitness	• Shoulders under water • Hips level and facing forward • Abdominals pulled in • Baby-bump lifted • Place heels down	• E: Smaller side steps • H: Larger side steps • E: March instead of shuffle • H: More spring on shuffles
Block 2 Knee lift on the spot Jog forwards Knee lift on the spot Jog back Repeat			• E: Narrower stance for the feet • H: Deeper squats • E: Smaller range of movement • H: Larger range of movement
Block 3 Squat on the spot Alternate arm pushes with closed fingers Repeat			• E: Shallower squats • H: Deeper squats • E: Slice hands through the water on arm push • E: Open the fingers for arm push • H: Speed up the arm movement or push both arms forward together instead of alternating the arms
Jog in a circle around the pool for active rest time THEN: Repeat all blocks once or twice			• E: March or jog on the spot • H: Faster jog or higher knees

PRENATAL MAIN ACTIVITY 3 – MIXED MUSCLE TONING AND CARDIOVASCULAR

Table 12.7	Prenatal main activity workout 3 – mixed muscle toning and cardiovascular		
Exercises	**Purpose**	**Teaching points**	**Alternatives**
Posture reinforcement			
Block 1 Jog forwards and squat on the spot x 10–15 reps Jog back and squat on the spot x 10–15 reps Repeat twice	To improve muscle tone and cardiovascular/ aerobic fitness	• Shoulders underwater • Hips level and facing forward • Abdominals pulled in • Baby-bump lifted • Place heels down on landing	• E: March instead of jog • H: More spring on shuffles • E: Narrower stance for the feet • H: Deeper squats
Block 2 Jog forwards Wall press x 8–10 reps 2 sets Jog back Leg curls on spot Side steps x 4 R Leg curls on the spot Side steps x 4 L Repeat twice			• E: Smaller range of movement • H: Larger range of movement
Block 3 Jog forwards Flutter kicks at pool wall x 10–15 reps, 2 sets Jacks on the spot Shuffles on the spot Repeat twice			• E: Walk forwards • E: Lower kicks • H: Higher kicks • E: Squats instead of jacks • H: More spring on jacks
Jog to pool wall Seated balance and pelvic floor exercises around the pool for active rest time THEN: Repeat all blocks once or twice			• E: March or jog on the spot • H: Faster jog or higher knees

PRENATAL MAIN ACTIVITY 4 – MIXED MUSCLE TONING AND CARDIOVASCULAR

Table 12.8	Prenatal main activity workout 3 – mixed muscle toning and cardiovascular		
Exercises	**Purpose**	**Teaching points**	**Alternatives**
Posture reinforcement			
Circuit station 1 Posture push	To improve muscle tone and cardiovascular/ aerobic fitness	• Shoulders underwater, brace abdominals • Hips forward, heels down	• E: Perform without float with arms extended in front of body and palms forward • H: Increase speed
Circuit station 2 Pool wall press-up		• Keep elbows slightly bent as arms straighten • Keep the baby-bump lifted throughout the movement	• E: Smaller movement • H: Triceps dips
Circuit station 3 Leg curl		• Keep heels down and shoulders underwater • Keep baby-bump pulled in and hips facing forward	• E: Smaller curl • E: Jog • H: Add a spring as legs change
Circuit station 4 Seated balance		• Keep back and neck long, ribcage lifted • Avoid holding the breath • Scull with hands for stability	• E: Use wall for added support • H: Keep one hand still in lap
Circuit station 5 Push/pull		• Shoulders underwater, brace abdominals • Hips forward, heels down • Try not to lock out elbows as arms are extended	• E: Perform without a partner • E: Perform with a partner but without a noodle and palms together • H: Increase resistance to the partner's movement
Circuit station 6 Low kick to the front		• Keep kicks low, knees bent • Abdominals and baby-bump tucked in • Heels down	• E: Less spring, knee lifts • H: More spring

PRENATAL COOL DOWNS
COOL DOWN 1

Table 12.9	Prenatal cool down 1		
Exercises	**Purpose**	**Teaching points**	**Alternatives**
Jogging in large circle around the pool	Cardiovascular/ aerobic	• Shoulders underwater • Hips level and facing forward • Baby-bump lifted • Place heels down	• E: March on the spot • H: High knees jog • Slower participants jog on the inside, faster participants on outside of the circle
Squats	Cardiovascular/ aerobic	• Shoulders underwater • Abdominals pulled in	• E: Smaller range of movement • H: Larger range of movement
Knee lifts	Cardiovascular/ aerobic	• Hips, knees and toes all in line • Keep heels down and shoulders underwater	• E: Smaller lifts • H: Bigger moves • H: Add a spring • If baby-bump is large, reduce height of knee lift or take knee slightly out to the side
Side steps R and L	Cardiovascular/ aerobic	• Shoulders underwater • Hips, knees and toes all in line • Baby-bump lifted and facing forward • Heels down	• E: Smaller side steps • E: Shallower squats • H: Faster side steps • H: Deeper squats
Repeat twice	Aim to decrease range of movement slightly to lower intensity and heart rate		

Table 12.9 Prenatal cool down 1 (cont.)

STRETCHES

Hamstring stretch	Static stretch for hamstrings	• Hips, knees and toes all in line • Keep heels down on the standing leg and shoulders underwater • Keep baby-bump lifted and hips level	• E: Lower leg lift • H: Higher leg lift, but keep hips level
Calf stretch	Static stretch for calf	• Shoulders underwater, baby-bump lifted and facing forward • Hips forward, heels down • Weight should be evenly distributed through both legs	• E: Narrower stance • H: Wider stance
Jog on the spot		• Shoulders underwater, abdominals in, hips and baby-bump facing forward • Heels down • Keep head up	• E: March
Squats	Cardiovascular/ aerobic	• Shoulders underwater • Abdominals pulled in	• E: Smaller range of movement • H: Larger range of movement
Pectoral stretch/ Breaststroke arms	Dynamic stretch for pectorals	• Shoulders underwater, brace abdominals • Hips forward, heels down • Fingers together	• E: Slice hands through the water with a flat hand • E: Open the fingers • H: Cup hands
Jog on the spot and stretch triceps	Triceps stretch (moving to keep warm)	• Shoulders underwater, abdominals in, hips and baby-bump facing forward • Heels down • Keep head up	• E: Elbow lower • H: Greater range of stretch

Table 12.9	Prenatal cool down 1 (cont.)		
Arm sweeps up and down (Tai chi style, see p. 101)	Dynamic stretch for the upper body	• Shoulders underwater • Abdominals pulled in	• E: Smaller range of movement • H: Larger range of movement
Single arm sweep across (Tai chi style, see p. 101)	Dynamic stretch for the upper body	• Shoulders underwater • Abdominals pulled in	• E: Smaller range of movement • H: Larger range of movement
Float on back with noodle support – pelvic floor contractions	Relaxation	• Allow the body to relax on the noodle	• E: Two noodles
Float on back with noodle support – focus on breathing	Relaxation	• Allow the body to relax on the noodle	• E: Two noodles

COOL DOWN 2

Table 12.10	Prenatal cool down 2		
Exercises	**Purpose**	**Teaching points**	**Alternatives**
Star jumps	Cardiovascular/ aerobic	• Shoulders underwater • Hips level and facing forward • Baby-bump lifted • Place heels down	• E: March on the spot • H: High knees jog
Knee lifts	Cardiovascular/ aerobic	• Hips, knees and toes all in line • Keep heels down and shoulders underwater	• E: Smaller lifts • H: Bigger moves • H: Add a spring • If baby-bump is large, reduce height of knee lift or take knee slightly out to the side

Table 12.10   Prenatal cool down 2 (cont.)

Jog forwards and march on the spot	Mobilising knees, ankles and hips and pulse raising	• Shoulders underwater, hips and baby-bump facing forward • Heels down	• E: Stay on the spot and jog/march • H: Lift knees higher, travel further
Jog backwards and march on the spot	Mobilising knees, ankles and hips and pulse raising	• Shoulders underwater, hips and baby-bump facing forward • Heels down	• E: Stay on the spot and jog/march • H: Lift knees higher, travel further
Repeat twice	Aim to decrease range of movement slightly to lower intensity and heart rate		

STRETCHES

Calf stretch	Static stretch for calf	• Shoulders underwater, baby-bump lifted and facing forwards • Hips forward, heels down • Weight should be evenly distributed through both legs	• E: Narrower stance • H: Wider stance
Pectoral stretch/ Breaststroke arms	Dynamic stretch for pectorals	• Shoulders underwater, brace abdominals • Hips forward, heels down • Fingers together	• E: Slice hands through the water with a flat hand • E: Open the fingers • H: Cup hands
Hamstring stretch	Static stretch for hamstrings	• Hips, knees and toes all in line • Keep heels down on the standing leg and shoulders underwater • Keep baby-bump lifted and hips level	• E: Lower leg lift • H: Higher leg lift, but keep hips level

Table 12.10	Prenatal cool down 2 (cont.)		
Squats	Cardiovascular/ aerobic	• Shoulders underwater • Abdominals pulled in	• E: Smaller range of movement • H: Larger range of movement • Slower participants jog on the inside, faster participants on outside of the circle
Jog in a circle and stretch triceps	Pulse lowering and triceps stretch	• Shoulders underwater, abdominals in, hips and baby-bump facing forward • Heels down • Keep head up	• E: Elbow lower • H: Greater range of stretch
Standing pelvic floor contractions and breathing focus	Strengthen pelvic floor	• Keep the arms moving gently	• E: Hold the side

SAMPLE FULL AQUA-NATAL CLASS

Table 12.11	Sample prenatal aqua class with timings		
Activity	**Purpose**	**Teaching points**	**Adaptations**
Welcome and Pre Screen Participants			
WARM–UP – mobility and pulse raising (5–6 minutes)			
Jogging in large circle around the pool	Pulse raising	• Shoulders underwater, hips and baby-bump facing forward • Heels down	Slower participants on the inside, faster participants on outside of the circle
Single arm sweeps across body (Tai chi, 'soothing')	Mobilising shoulders	Back straight, baby-bump tucked in, fingers together, hands cupped	Keep arm a bit bent, open fingers
Shallow squats	Mobilising knees and hips and pulse raising	• Hips, knees and toes all in line • Baby-bump facing forward • Heels down • Shoulders underwater	Shallower knee bends if preferred
Arm sweeps forward and back on the spot (Tai chi, style p. 101)	Mobilising shoulders	• Shoulders underwater, hips forward, heels down • Fingers together, hands cupped	Reduce or increase range of movement
Side steps R and squat Repeat to L	Mobilising hips and knees/pulse raising	• Shoulders underwater, brace abdominals • Hips forward, heels down • Arms pull across body opposite to direction of travel • Fingers together, hands cupped	Jog on spot if preferred
Knee lifts	Mobilising hips and knees/pulse raising	• Hips, knees and toes all in line • Keep heels down and shoulders underwater	Reduce range of movement or jog on the spot if preferred
Repeat from SQUATS			

AQUA EXERCISE

Table 12.11	**Sample prenatal aqua class with timings (cont.)**		
WARM-UP PREP STRETCH – static or dynamic stretches (3–4 minutes)			
Hamstring stretch	Static stretch for hamstrings	• Hips, knees and toes all in line • Keep heels down and shoulders underwater • Keep baby-bump lifted	Offer support of the pool wall for static stretches: Calf, hamstring, inner thigh
Calf stretch	Static stretch for calf	• Shoulders underwater, baby-bump lifted • Hips forward, heels down	Reduce width of stance if discomfort in pelvis
Breaststroke arms	Dynamic stretch for pectorals	• Shoulders underwater, brace abdominals • Hips forward, heels down • Fingers together	Open fingers to reduce resistance
Jog on the spot and stretch triceps	Stretch triceps, keep moving and warm	• Shoulders underwater, abdominals in, hips and baby-bump facing forward • Heels down and head up	March in place
Inner thigh stretch	Static stretch for adductors	• Shoulders underwater, brace abdominals, baby-bump lifted • Hips forward, heels down • Knees and toes in line	Reduce width of stretch if discomfort in pelvis
Squats on the spot	Keep moving and warm	As before	As before
RE-WARM (4 mins)			
Side steps R	Cardiovascular /aerobic	• Shoulders underwater, hips forward, baby-bump tucked in, heels down • Arms underwater, sweep opposite to direction of travel • Fingers together, hands cupped	• Reduce range of movement if discomfort in pelvis • Jog forward to R if preferred

Table 12.11   Sample prenatal aqua class with timings (cont.)

Squats Repeat all L	Cardiovascular /aerobic	As before	As before
Jog forwards	Cardiovascular /aerobic	Abdominals tucked in, baby-bump lifted and facing forward, hips and shoulders facing forward, heels down	Walk forwards if preferred
Leg kicks on the spot	Cardiovascular /aerobic	• Keep kicks low, knees bent • Abdominals and baby-bump tucked in • Heels down	Knee lift on the spot if preferred
Jog back and leg kicks on the spot	Cardiovascular /aerobic	As before	Walk backwards if preferred
Repeat from side steps – aim to increase ROM to increase intensity and heart rate			

MAIN CIRCUIT-STYLE WORKOUT
(1 min work: 30 secs rest. Twice round = 18 mins total)
*Encourage group to work in pairs and socialise

Water walking	Strength/ endurance for postural and leg muscles Also cardiovascular	*Opportunity for education about good posture	Hold arms in front, palms forward for added resistance
Wall press	Strength/ endurance for triceps and pectorals	Keep elbows slightly bent as arms straighten	Reduce range of movement
Seated balance	Strength/ endurance for deep abdominal muscles	*Opportunity for education about seated posture	Use wall for support if balance is difficult

Table 12.11	Sample prenatal aqua class with timings (cont.)		
Leg kicks on the spot	Cardiovascular	See p. 144	Jog on the spot
Breaststroke arm sweeps	Strength/ endurance for pectorals and trapezius	See p. 143	• Fingers closed, hands cupped to add resistance • Fingers open for less resistance • Use wall for support
Travelling leg lunges	Cardiovascular and strength/ endurance for quadriceps and gluteals	Static lunges	

COOL DOWN – Lowering the pulse (3–4 minutes)

Jogging in large circle around pool	CV/aerobic	As before	As before
Squats	CV/aerobic	As before	Shallower squat if preferred
Knee lifts	CV/aerobic	As before	Jog on the spot
Side steps R and L	CV/aerobic	As before	As before

Repeat all, but reduce range of movement to reduce intensity and heart rate

COOL DOWN – Stretch and relaxation, static or dynamic stretches (5–7 minutes)

Quads stretch	Static stretch	As before	Offer support of the wall for any stretch requiring balance, e.g. quads
Hamstrings stretch	Static stretch		
Calf stretch	Static stretch		
Jog on the spot	Warming		
Squats	Warming		
Breaststroke arms	Dynamic stretch		

Table 12.11 Sample prenatal aqua class with timings (cont.)

Triceps stretch	Static stretch	As before	Offer support of the wall for any stretch requiring balance, e.g. quads
Inner thigh stretch	Static stretch		
Arm sweeps up and down	Remobilise shoulders		
Single arm sweeps across	Remobilise shoulders		
Float on back with noodle support – pelvic floor contractions	Relaxation* Strengthen pelvic floor**	* Opportunity to practise techniques in preparation for labour **Opportunity for education about pelvic floor	
Float on back with noodle support – effleurage	Relaxation*		

Table 12.12 Sample postnatal session using equipment

Activity	Purpose	Teaching points	Adaptations
Pre Screen Participants			
WARM–UP (5–6 minutes)			
Jogging in large circle around the pool	Pulse raising/ warming	• Shoulders underwater, abdominals in, hips facing forward • Heels down	Slower participants jog on inside, faster participants on outside of the circle
Breaststroke arms	Mobilising shoulders	Back straight, tummy tucked in, fingers together, hands cupped	Keep arm a bit bent, open fingers
Leg curls	Mobilising knees and hips and pulse raising	• Hips, knees and toes all in line • Pelvis facing forwards • Heels down • Shoulders underwater	Squat if preferred

Table 12.13	Sample postnatal session using equipment (cont.)		
Double arm sweep with a trunks twist	Mobilising shoulders and spine	• Shoulders underwater, brace abdominals • Hips forward, heels down • Fingers together, hands cupped	Reduce or increase range of movement
Side steps R and squat Repeat to L	Mobilising hips and knees/pulse raising	• Shoulders underwater, brace abdominals • Hips forward, heels down • Arms pull across body opposite to direction of travel • Fingers together, hands cupped	Narrower steps if preferred
Jacks	Mobilising hips and knees/pulse raising	• Shoulders underwater, brace abdominals • Knees and toes in line • Heels down on landing	Reduce range of movement or jog on the spot if preferred

Repeat from LEG CURLS

PREP STRETCH – static or dynamic stretches (3–4 minutes)

Hamstring stretch	Static stretch for hamstrings	• Hips, knees and toes all in line • Keep heels down and shoulders underwater • Brace abdominals	Offer support of the pool wall for static stretches: Calf, hamstring, inner thigh
Calf stretch	Static stretch for calf	• Shoulders underwater, brace abdominals, baby-bump lifted • Hips forward, heels down	Reduce width of stance if discomfort in pelvis
Breaststroke arms	Dynamic stretch for pectorals	• Shoulders underwater, brace abdominals • Hips forward, heels down • Fingers together	Open fingers to reduce resistance
Jog on the spot and stretch triceps	Stretch triceps while keeping moving and warm	• Shoulders underwater, abdominals in, hips and baby-bump facing forward • Heels down • Keep head up	Leave out jogging

Table 12.13	Sample postnatal session using equipment (cont.)		
Side leg kicks	Dynamic stretch for adductors	• Shoulders underwater, brace abdominals, baby-bump lifted • Hips forward, heels down • Knees and toes in line	Static stretch if discomfort is felt in pelvis
Jacks	Keep moving and warm	As before	Squats on the spot
RE-WARM (4 mins)			
Side gallops R	CV/aerobic	• Shoulders underwater, hips forward, pelvis tucked in, heels down • Arms underwater, sweep opposite to direction of travel • Fingers together, hands cupped	Reduce range of movement if discomfort in pelvis. Jog forward to R if preferred
Shuffle Repeat all L	CV/aerobic	• Hips and shoulders forward • Shoulders underwater	As before
Fast jog on the spot	CV/aerobic	• Abdominals tucked in, hips and shoulders facing forwards, • Heels down	Squat if preferred
Power knee lifts on the spot	CV/aerobic	• Abdominals tucked in • Heels down, knees soft on landing	Knee lift on the spot if preferred
Fast jog on the spot	CV/aerobic	As above	Walk backwards if preferred
Repeat from Side Gallops – aim to increase ROM to increase intensity and heart rate			
MAIN CIRCUIT-STYLE WORKOUT **(1 min work: 30 secs rest. Twice round circuit = 18 mins total)** *Encourage group to work in pairs and socialise			
Aqua jog	Cardiovascular	• Abdominals in, hips forward • Heels down	With or without the noodle for added resistance

| Table 12.13 | Sample postnatal session using equipment (cont.) |

Pec flyes	Strength/ endurance for pectorals and trapezius	• Shoulders underwater, abdominals in, hips facing forward	Reduce range of movement
Abdominal leg sweeps	Strength/ endurance for transverse abdominals and rectus abdominis	• Brace abdominals • Keep feet and knees together	• Use wall or float for support • Keep knees bent and tuck in
Vertical jumps	Cardiovascular	Knees bent and heels down on landing	Jog on the spot
Pushdowns with float	Strength/ endurance for triceps and shoulders	Shoulders underwater, abdominals in, hips facing forward	With/without noodle for added resistance
Bent leg twists	Strength/ endurance for obliques	• Brace abdominals • Keep feet and knees together	Use wall for support

COOL DOWN (3–4 minutes)

Jogging in large circle around pool	CV/aerobic	As before	As before
Jacks	CV/aerobic	As before	Squat if preferred
Leg curls	CV/aerobic	As before	Jog on the spot
Side steps R and L	CV/aerobic	As before	As before

Repeat all, but reduce range of movement to reduce intensity and heart rate

COOL DOWN STRETCH AND RELAXATION (5–7 minutes): static or dynamic stretches

Quads stretch	Static stretch to re-lengthen quads	As before	Offer support of the wall for any stretch requiring balance, e.g. quads

Table 12.13 Sample postnatal session using equipment (cont.)			
Hamstring stretch	Static stretch to re-lengthen hamstrings	As before	As before
Calf stretch	Static stretch to re-lengthen calf		
Jog on the spot	Warming		
Knee lifts	Warming		
Breaststroke arms	Dynamic (moving) stretch for pectorals		
Triceps stretch	Static stretch to re-lengthen triceps		
Side leg kicks	Dynamic stretch for adductors		
Arm sweeps up and down	Remobilise shoulders		
Single arm sweeps across	Remobilise shoulders		
Float on back with noodle support – pelvic floor contractions	• Relaxation • Strengthen pelvic floor		

RECOMMENDED READING
AND INFORMATION SOURCES

Clapp, J. F., *Exercising Through Your Pregnancy* (Addicus Books 2002)

Coulson M., and Bolitho, S., *The Complete Guide to Pregnancy and Fitness* (Bloomsbury 2012)

DiFiore, J., *The Complete Guide to Postnatal Fitness* (A & C Black 2003)

Rankin, J., *Effects of Antenatal Exercise on Psychological Well-being, Pregnancy and Birth Outcome* (Whurr Publishers 2002)

American Congress of Obstetricians and Gynecologists
www.acog.org

Royal College of Obstetricians and Gynaecologists
www.rcog.org.uk

Royal College of Midwives
www.rcm.org.uk

The Association of Chartered Physiotherapists in Women's Health
www.womensphysio.com

APPENDIX 1 – EXERCISE GUIDELINES

Early Years (under 5s)

- Physical activity should be encouraged from birth, particularly through floor-based play and water-based activities in safe environments

- Children of pre-school age who are capable of walking unaided should be physically active daily for at least 180 minutes (3 hours), spread throughout the day

- All under 5s should minimise the amount of time spent being sedentary (being restrained or sitting) for extended periods (except time spent sleeping)

Children and Young People (5–18 years)

- All children and young people should engage in moderate to vigorous intensity physical activity for at least 60 minutes and up to several hours every day

- Vigorous intensity activity, including those activities that strengthen muscle and bone, should be incorporated at least 3 days a week

- All children and young people should minimise the time spent being sedentary (sitting) for extended periods

Adults (19–64 years)

- Adults should aim to be active daily. Over a week, activity should add up to at least 150 minutes (2½ hours) of moderate intensity activity in bouts of 10 minutes or more – one way to approach this is to do 30 minutes on at least five days per week

- Alternatively comparable benefits can be achieved through 75 minutes of vigorous activity spread across the week or a moderate and vigorous intensity activity

- Adults should also undertake activity to improve muscle strength on at least two days a week

- All adults should minimise the time spent being sedentary (sitting) for extended periods

Older Adults (over 65+ years)

- Older adults who participate in any physical activity gain some health benefits, including maintenance of good physical and cognitive function. Some physical activity is better than none and more physical activity provides greater health benefits

- Older adults should aim to be active daily. Over a week, activity should add up to at least 150 minutes (2½) hours) of moderate intensity activity in bouts of 10 minutes or more – one way to approach this is to do 30 minutes on at least five days per week

- For those who are already active at moderate intensity, comparable benefits can be achieved through 75 minutes of vigorous activity spread across the week or a moderate and vigorous intensity activity

- Older adults at risk of falls should incorporate physical activity to improve balance and co-ordination on at least two days per week

- All older adults should minimise the time spent being sedentary (sitting) for extended periods

Source: *Start Active, Stay Active*, NHS 2011

TRIMESTER ONE (WEEKS 1–13 APPROX)

Many of the anatomical and physiological changes of pregnancy will not be very evident in the 1st trimester and if the woman is a regular exerciser and does not have any medical issues there is no reason why she cannot continue as normal. That said, now is not the time to work on improving fitness – a maintenance programme is much more appropriate and safer too.

The 1st trimester is a good time to lay the groundwork for good posture, alignment and technique for the coming 8–9 months. New exercises can also be practised (if mum-to-be is not already doing them) in order to minimise the impact of pregnancy related changes later.

Published recommendations from ACOG:

In the absence of any contra-indications, 30 minutes or more of moderate exercise on most, if not all, days of the week. (Always check with health professional first.)

After 1st trimester, avoid supine positions during exercise and motionless standing.

Avoid activities with a high risk of falling or abdominal trauma, for example ice hockey, football.

Scuba diving only under doctor's direction.

Exertions at altitudes up to 6000ft appear safe. Higher altitudes carry a risk of hypoxemia.

TRIMESTER TWO (WEEKS 14–27 APPROX)

The 2nd trimester may be when the physiological and anatomical changes of pregnancy begin to affect the woman and become obvious to others. Specific adaptations will need to be made to her programme in terms of intensity and type of activities included.

Published recommendations from ACOG, RCOG, ACPWH (The Association of Chartered Physiotherapists in Women's Health), CSEP (Canadian Society for Exercise Physiology), SCOG (Society of Obstetricians and Gynaecologists of Canada), ACSM (American College of Sports Medicine), RACOG (Royal Australian College of Obstetricians and Gynaecologists) relevant to 2nd trimester and the rest of pregnancy:

Avoid supine lying (lying on back) from weeks 16–20 onwards due to the risk of supine hypotensive syndrome.

TRIMESTER THREE (WEEKS 28–40/42 APPROX)

The 3rd trimester is a time when the woman may really be feeling the effects of her pregnancy. There is lots of additional weight placing stress on her back and joints, making her feel tired, not to mention the squashing of her internal organs! The mother may also be starting to get anxious about labour and delivery.

It is now appropriate to really taper intensity down and focus on maintaining mobility and posture as far as possible. It is also a good time to give some tips on appropriate activity for the immediate postnatal period, especially pelvic floor and abdominals.

THE IMMEDIATE POSTNATAL PERIOD

Exercise in the immediate postnatal period (0–6 weeks post-partum) should be gentle and gradual with a focus on daily activity rather than exercise. Recommended activities include:

- Walking
- Abdominal hollowing
- Pelvic tilts
- Pelvic floor exercises

Absolute contraindications – Conditions or circumstances where exercise is contra-indicated.

Aerobic fitness – The ability to deliver oxygen to the working muscles and use it during exercise.

Afterbirth – A collective term for the placenta, umbilical cord and amniotic sac/membranes, usually delivered a few minutes or hours after the baby.

Agility – A rapid whole-body movement with change of velocity or direction in response to a stimulus.

Agonist – Refers to a muscle or muscle group responsible for the main action.

Air embolism – An air bubble that becomes trapped in a blood vessel.

Alpha fetoprotein – A protein produced by the foetus. AFP testing may be done to check the foetus for certain conditions such as spina bifida or liver disorders.

Amniocentesis – A process involving withdrawal of a sample of amniotic fluid for the purpose of testing for chromosomal abnormalities and other conditions.

Amnion – The membrane in which the foetus develops.

Amniotic fluid – The fluid that surrounds the foetus in the uterus.

Antagonist – Refers to a muscle or muscle group responsible for opposing the main action.

Apgar score – Assessment of baby immediately after birth. Named after Virginia Apgar.

Aponeurosis – A fibrous sheet of tissue to which muscles attach instead of to tendons. Abdominal aponeurosis connects abdominal muscles to the linea alba.

Areola – Area of pigmentation surrounding the nipple.

Arrhythmia – Deviation from normal heartbeat.

ASIS – The anterior superior iliac spine, often called the 'hip bones'.

Asthma – Type of obstructive lung disease.

Baroreceptor – A sensory nerve ending that responds to changes in blood pressure.

Blood pressure – The force of the blood on the artery walls.

BMI – Body mass index (weight in kilograms divided by height in metres squared).

Bradycardia – Low resting heart rate.

Braxton Hicks contractions – 'Practice' contractions occurring in pregnancy, usually becoming stronger towards term.

Breech presentation – Where the foetus is lying feet or bottom down; occurs in approximately 4% of pregnancies.

Calorie – The amount of energy needed to increase the temperature of 1 gram of water by 1°C.

Cardiac output – The amount of blood pumped out of each ventricle per minute.

Carpal tunnel syndrome – Compression of the medial nerve in the wrist leading to tingling or numbness in the thumb, index and middle fingers.

Cell – Basic structural and functional unit of life.

Centre of gravity – The point at which the body can be balanced.

Cerclage – A procedure where an incompetent cervix is closed with a stitch/suture to avoid opening under pressure during pregnancy.

Chemoreceptor – A cell that responds to levels of chemicals in the body.

Chorionic villus sampling – This involves a sample of placental cells being removed and tested for genetic defects.

Collagen – The key component of all connective tissue.

Colostrum – Fluid breast secretions occurring in late pregnancy and after delivery. Also called 'first milk'.

Conception – Fertilisation of egg signalling the start of pregnancy.

Congenital – Term used to describe a condition that was present at birth.

Contraction – Shortening of muscle fibres due to electrical stimulation.

Corpus luteum – The outer covering of ovarian follicle.

Delayed onset muscle soreness – Perception of post-exercise soreness.

Developmental stretch – A stretch held long enough to induce physical structure development to increase flexibility.

Diastasis recti – The separation of the linea alba in/following pregnancy.

Diastolic – The relaxation phase of the heart beat cycle.

Dilation/dilatation – The enlargement or widening of the cervix.

Doming – A bulge occurring in the abdomen when rectus abdominis is contracted, particularly when diastasis recti is present.

Down's Syndrome – A condition resulting from chromosomal abnormality.

Dual concentric contraction – A movement in which both muscles in a pair contract in order to bring about a movement.

Dyspnoea – Shortness of breath.

Ectopic pregnancy – The implantation of a fertilised egg outside the uterus.

Eddy current – A current that flows in water, opposite the normal flow.

Endocrine system – An integrated system of organs, glands and tissues that involve the release of extracellular signalling molecules known as hormones.

Endometrium – The lining of the uterine wall.

Enzymes – Proteins that can speed up chemical reactions.

Epidural – A type of anaesthesia used during labour/birth.

Episiotomy – An incision/cut of the perineum performed to facilitate childbirth.

Erythrocyte – A red blood cell.

Expected Delivery Date – The anticipated date of delivery.

Extension – Movement at a joint in which the joint angle increases.

Fallopian tube – A tube connecting the ovary to the uterus.

Flexibility – The available range of motion around a specific joint.

Flexion – Movement at a joint in which the joint angle decreases.

Foetus – The developing baby in the uterus.

Forceps – Specially designed tongs used to assist birth.

Fundus – The top of the uterus, the fundal height is a measurement taken from the top of the pubic bone to the fundus and is used to estimate the growth of the foetus.

Gestation – The period of pregnancy.

Gestational diabetes – Impaired glucose tolerance or diabetes occurring during pregnancy.

Gestational hypertension – see pregnancy induced hypertension.

Gland – A group of cells that release hormones.

Haemodynamically significant – Haemodynamic relates to the circulation of blood, in particular blood pressure and haemodynamically significant means that there is a considerable effect on blood circulation.

Haemoglobin – Part of a red blood cell that carries oxygen or carbon dioxide.

Haemorrhoids – Varicose veins occurring in the anus, also known as piles.

Heart rate – The number of heart beats per minute.

Histamine – A chemical in the body that has the effect of widening the airways.

Homeostasis – When the systems of the body are working optimally and within set limits.

Hormone – A chemical messenger in the body.

Human Chorionic Gonadotropin – Hormone produced in pregnancy, maintains production of progesterone.

Hydrostatic pressure – The pressure of water on the submerged body.

Hyperemesis/hyperemesis gravidarum – Severe or extreme nausea and/or vomiting during pregnancy.

Hyperglycaemia – High levels of blood glucose.

Hypertension – High blood pressure.

Hypertrophy – Enlargement of an organ such as a muscle.

Hypoglycaemia – Low levels of blood glucose.

Hypotension – Low blood pressure.

Hypothermia – A body temperature of below 34 or 35°C.

Hypoxia – Reduced oxygen supply to tissues.

Incompetent cervix – When the cervix is unable to remain closed during pregnancy; can increase risk of second trimester miscarriage.

Induction – When labour is started artificially.

Insulin – A hormone secreted by the pancreas, involved in the regulation of blood sugar levels.

Intensity – A measurement of the difficulty level or 'hardness' of the exercise.

Intrauterine growth restriction (IUGR) – Where the foetus does not grow in line with expected potential. Also called 'small for dates'.

In utero – Inside the uterus.

Ischaemia – A low oxygen state (normally due to blocked arteries).

IVF/In vitro fertilisation – The process by which an egg is fertilised outside the body then implanted into the uterus.

Kegel exercises – Exercise designed to tone the pelvic floor muscles.

Kyphosis – Curvature of the thoracic spine.

Labour – The term given to the process of delivery of baby and afterbirth from the uterus.

Lactation – The secretion of milk from the breasts.

Lightening – When the baby moves down into the pelvis in preparation for birth, also called 'dropping' or 'engaging'.

Linea alba – A band of tendon occurring at the aponeurosis of the abdominal muscles.

Linea negra – A dark line that develops along the linea alba during pregnancy.

LMP/Last menstrual period – Used to date the pregnancy.

Lordosis – Excessive primary curve of the lumbar spine.

Macrosomia – An abnormally large foetus.

Mastitis – An inflammation of the breast often occurring while breastfeeding.

Maximum heart rate (MHR) – Theoretically the maximum possible heart rate for an individual.

Metabolic equivalent (MET) – A method of expressing energy expenditure.

Metabolic rate – The amount of energy expended at a given time.

Metabolic syndrome – A combination of abdominal obesity, hypertension, dyslipidemia and impaired fasting glucose.

Miscarriage – Loss of the foetus before 20 weeks of pregnancy. Most common in weeks 8–12. Also known as Spontaneous Miscarriage or Spontaneous Abortion.

Multiparity – Second or subsequent pregnancies or carrying more than one foetus.

Multiple gestation – A pregnancy with more than one foetus, twins, triplets etc.

Muscular endurance – The ability of a muscle or muscle group to perform repeated contractions against a resistance over a period of time.

Muscular strength – The maximum amount of force a muscle or muscle group can generate.

Neural – Relating to the nervous system.

Neuromuscular – Relating to the muscular and associated nervous system.

Nipple – Protruding structure in the middle of the breast, surrounded by the areola.

Noradrenaline – A stress hormone (also known as norepinephrine).

Obesity – The percentage of body fat at which the risk of disease to the individual is increased.

Obstructive lung disease – A condition/s where damage to the lungs or airways cause difficulty with expiration.

Oestrogen – Steroid hormone, key to female sexual development, responsible for growth of foetus and breasts in pregnancy.

Omphalocele – Term used to describe a birth defect in which the baby's intestines or other abdominal organs protrude out of the navel.

Ovary – The female reproductive organ that is responsible for production of eggs and hormones.

Ovulation – Release of mature egg (ovum) from an ovary.

Oxytocin – A hormone that stimulates contractions in labour and milk production after birth.

Pancreas – Organ in the body that secretes insulin.

PAR-Q – Physical activity readiness questionnaire.

Perceived exertion – A subjective measurement of exercise intensity.

Perineum – The area between the vagina and the anus.

Pica – Craving or eating of non-food substances such as charcoal, paper etc.

Placenta – Uterine organ which attaches the embryo/foetus to the uterus and which provides nutrients and eliminates waste from the foetus.

Placental abruption – A condition where bleeding from the placenta leads to detachment of the placenta from the wall of the uterus. May be associated with hypertension and pre-eclampsia. Also called Abruptio Placentae.

Placenta praevia – A condition where the placenta is lying (fully or partly) over the lower part of the uterus, next to or covering the cervix.

Plasma – Major fluid component of blood in which blood cells are suspended.

Pregnancy Induced Hypertension – The development of raised blood pressure during pregnancy (also known as gestational hypertension).

Presyncope – A state of dizziness and/or weakness often preceding a faint.

Preterm – Relates to birth or rupture of membranes before 37 weeks.

Progesterone – A steroid hormone that prepares the endometrium for pregnancy, and relaxes smooth muscle tissue during pregnancy.

Prolactin – Hormone responsible for stimulating milk production after delivery and stimulation of progesterone.

Prone – Lying on the front.

Proprioceptive neuromuscular facilitation (PNF) – A type of stretching.

Proprioceptor – A sensory nerve ending that monitors position of the body.

Residual volume – The volume of air remaining in the lungs at the end of a maximal expiration.

Resting heart rate (RHR) – The heart rate at resting levels measured in beats per minute (bpm).

Restrictive lung disease – A condition/s where the lungs cannot fully expand thus restricting inspiration.

Round ligaments – The ligaments that support the uterus.

Rupture of membranes – The breaking of the amniotic sac, often referred to as 'waters breaking' and an indication that labour has started/ will start soon.

Scoliosis – Curvature of the spine.

Screening – A process used to determine health status.

Smooth muscle – Muscle found in the walls of hollow organs that is not under voluntary control.

Stability – A body's resistance to the disturbance of equilibrium.

Stillbirth – When there are no signs of life in a foetus after 24 weeks.

Stretch marks – Areas of stretched skin due to hormones and/or expanding abdomen.

Stretching – The method or technique used to influence the joint range of motion.

Stroke volume – The amount of blood ejected from one ventricle per heartbeat.

Subcutaneous – A layer of tissue lying just below the dermis layer.

Supine – Lying on the back.

Syncope – Loss of consciousness or fainting, often due to a fall in blood pressure.

Systolic – Maximum pressure on the artery walls during contraction of the left ventricle.

Tachycardia – High resting heart rate.

Tendon – Connective tissue that surrounds muscle fibres.

Termination – A medically directed termination of a pregnancy that can be legally carried out before 24 weeks. Also referred to as Abortion.

Testosterone – A steroid hormone that is responsible for muscle growth.

Thermoreceptor – A sensory nerve ending, responds to changes in temperature.

Thermoregulation – The regulation of temperature using various systems within the body.

Tidal volume – The volume of air that is inhaled or exhaled with each breath.

Transversus abdominis – Muscle of the core.

Umbilical cord – A cord-like tissue strand connecting the foetus and placenta.

Uterus – Pear shaped pelvic organ, site of implantation of fertilised egg (ovum).

Validity (test) – Purported to specifically measure what the tester or testing team is investigating.

Vasoconstriction – Narrowing of the lumen of blood vessels.

Vasodilation – Increase in size of lumen of blood vessels.

VO2max – Symbol for maximal oxygen consumption, the maximum amount of oxygen that can be delivered to the working muscles.

Womb – A term for the uterus.

APPENDIX 4 – REFERENCES

ACOG Committee Opinion, No. 267. 'Exercise during pregnancy and the postpartum period.' *Obstetrics and Gynaecology*, 99: 171–173

ACPWH (2004) *Aquanatal Guidelines* (Revised). Association of Chartered Physiotherapists in Women's Health

ACPWH (2005) 'Announcements from the Executive. Joint Statement' from: HACP (Hydrotherapy Association of Chartered Physiotherapists) and ACPWH (Association of Chartered Physiotherapists in Women's Health) March

Artal R. & Sherman C. (1999) 'Exercise during pregnancy.' *The Physician and Sports Medicine* 27

Becker, B. E. (2011) 'Biophysiologic aspects of hydrotherapy', in Cole, A.J., Becker B.E. eds. *Comprehensive Aquatic Therapy*, 3rd Edition. Washington: Washington State University Press; 19–56

Berk B. (2004) 'Recommending exercise during and after pregnancy: what the evidence says', *International Journal of Childbirth Education*, 19(2): 18–24.

Bø K. & Finckenhagen H. (2003) 'Is there any difference in measurement of pelvic floor muscle strength in supine and standing position?' *Acta Obstetricia et Gynecologica Scandinavica*, 82 (12): 1120–1124

Bolitho, S., Lawrence, D. & McNish, E., (2013) *The Complete Guide to Behavioural Change*, London: Bloomsbury

Borg, G. (1970) 'Perceived exertion as an indicator of somatic stress', *Scandinavian Journal of Rehabilitation Medicine*, 2: 92–98

Borg, G., (1982) 'A category scale with ratio properties for intermodal and inter-individual comparisons' in: Geissler, H.G., Petzold, P. eds. *Psychophysical judgement and the process of perception*, Berlin, VEB Deutscher Verlag der Wissenschaften, 25–34

Boscaglia, N., Skouteris, H., Wertheim, E.H., (2003) 'Changes in body image satisfaction during pregnancy: a comparison of high exercising and low exercising women', *Australia and New Zealand Journal of Obstetrics & Gynaecology*, 43(1): 41–45

CEMACH (2007) *The Confidential Enquiry into Maternal and Child Health*, 'Saving Mothers Lives: reviewing maternal deaths to make motherhood safer' (2003–2005)

Chief Medical Officer: At least five a week. Evidence on the impact of physical activity and its relationship to health (2004)

Clapp J., (2002), *Exercising Through Your Pregnancy*, Nebraskas: Addicus Books

Clapp J.F., *et al.* (2000) 'Beginning exercise in early pregnancy: effect on fetoplacental growth', *American Journal of Obstetrics and Gynaecology*, Dec; 183 (6): 14841488

Clapp, J., Kim, H., Burcui, B., (2002) 'Continuing regular exercise during pregnancy: effect of exercise volume on fetal placental growth', *American Journal of Obstetrics and Gynecology*, 1861:142–7

Claesson, I.M., Josefsson, A.,; Cedergren, *et al.*, (2008) 'Consumer satisfaction with a weight-gain intervention programme for obese pregnant women', *Midwifery*, June, 24 Issue: Number 2, p163–7

Dempsey, J.C., Butler, C.L., Williams, M.A., (2005) 'No need for a pregnancy pause: physical activity may reduce the occurrence of gestational diabetes mellitus and preeclampsia', *Exercise and Sports Science Reviews*, 33(3): 141–9.

DiNallo, J. M., Downs, D. S., (2007) 'The Role of Exercise in Preventing and Treating Gestational Diabetes: A Comprehensive Review and Recommendations for Future Research', *Journal of Applied Biobehavioral Research*, July, 12 Issue: p141–177

Duncombe, D., Wertheim, E.H., Skouteris H., *et al.* (2009) 'Factors related to exercise over the course of pregnancy including women's beliefs about the safety of exercise during pregnancy', *Midwifery*, 25(4): 430-8. Epub 2007, Dec 11

Durham, H.A., Morey, M.C., Lovelady, C.A., *et al.* (2011) 'Postpartum physical activity in overweight and obese women', *J Phys Act Health*, Sep 8 (7): 988

Evans, J., (2001) 'Cohort study of depressed mood during pregnancy and after childbirth', *British Medical Journal*, 323, pp. 257–260, Evidence Level 2+ (Cohort Study)

Evenson, K.R. & Wen, F., (2010) 'Measuring physical activity among pregnant women using a structured one-week recall questionnaire: evidence for validity and reliability', *Int. J Behav Nutr Phys Act*, Mar 21; 7:21

Fell, D.B., Joseph, K.S., Armson, B.A., *et al.* (2009) 'The Impact of Pregnancy on Physical Activity Level', *Maternal and Child Health Journal*, September, 13 Issue: Number 5 p597–603

Gaston, A., Cramp, A., (2011) 'Exercise during pregnancy: a review of patterns and determinants', July 14 (4):299–305. Epub: 2011 Mar 21

Greenleaf, J.E., (1984) 'Physiological responses to prolonged bed rest and fluid immersion in humans', *J Appl Physiol*, 57: 619–633

Haakstad, L.A., Voldner N., Bø K, (2013) 'Stages of change model for participation in physical activity during pregnancy', *J Pregnancy*, 193170. Epub: 2013 Feb 4

Haakstad, L.A., Voldner, N., Henriksen, T., Bø K, (2009) 'Why do pregnant women stop exercising in the third trimester?' *Acta Obstet Gynecol Scand*, 88(11):1267–75

Hartmann, S., Bung, P, (1999) 'Physical Exercise During Pregnancy – Physiological Considerations and Recommendations', *Journal of Perinatal Medicine*, 27 (3):204–215

Hatch, M., Levin, B., Shu–Xiao, O., *et al.* (1998) 'Maternal leisure time exercise and timely delivery', *American Journal of Public Health*, 88(1): 1528–1533

Hegaard, H.K., Pedersen, B.K., Nielsen, B.B., *et al.* (2007) 'Leisure time physical activity during pregnancy and impact on gestational diabetes mellitus, pre-eclampsia, preterm delivery and birth weight: a review', *Acta Obstetricia et Gynecologica Scandinavica*, 86(11):1290–1296

Huch, R. & Erkkola, R. (1990) 'Pregnancy and Exercise – Exercise and Pregnancy', *British Journal of Obstetrics and Gynaecology*, 61, pp705–9

Juhl, M., Madsen, M., Andersen, A.M.N., *et al.* (2012) 'Distribution and predictors of exercise habits among pregnant women in the Danish National Birth Cohort', *Scandinavian Journal of Medicine & Science in Sports*, February, 22 Issue: Number 1 p128–138

Katz, V.L., (2003) 'Exercise in Water During Pregnancy', *Clinical Obstetrics and Gynaecology*, 46:432–441

Katz, V.L., (1996) 'Water Exercise in Pregnancy', *Seminars in Perinatology*, 20:285-291

Katz, V., McMurray R., Goodwin W., *et al.* (1990) 'Nonweightbearing Exercise During Pregnancy on Land and During Immersion: A Comparative Study', *American Journal of Perinatology*, July, 7 Issue: Number 3 p281–4

Kent, T., Gregor, J., Leardorff, L., Katz, V., (1999) 'Edema of Pregnancy: A comparison of water aerobics and static immersion', *Obstetrics & Gynaecology* 94; 5

Kihlstrand, M., Stenman, B., Nilsson, S., *et al.* (1999) 'Water Gymnastics Reduced the Intensity of Back/Low Back Pain in Pregnant Women', *Acta Obstetricia Gynecologica Scandinavica*, 78:180–5

Kim, K., Chung, E., Kim C., *et al.* (2012) 'Swimming exercise during pregnancy alleviates pregnancy-associated long-term memory impairment', *Physiology & Behavior*, August, vol 107, Issue: 1, p.82–86

Lawrence, D., (2004) *The Complete Guide to Exercise in Water*, 2nd Edition, London: A&C Black

Lox, C.L., Treasure, D.C., 'Changes in feeling states following aquatic exercise during pregnancy', (2000) *Journal of Applied Social Psychology*, 30 (3): 518–527

May, L. M., (2008) 'Labor of love: Physically active moms-to-be give babies a head start on heart health', presented at *Federation of American Societies for Experimental Biology* 2011

McMurray, R.G., Hackney, A.C., Guion, W.K., *et al.* (1996) 'Metabolic and hormonal responses to low-impact aerobic dance during pregnancy', *Clinical Sciences,* 28(1): 41-46

Medforth, J., Battersby, S., Evans, M., *et al.* (2006) *Oxford Handbook of Midwifery*, Oxford: Oxford University Press

Merati, G., Rampichini, S., Roselli, M., *et al.* (2006) 'Gravity and gravidity: will microgravity assist pregnancy?' *Sport Sciences for Health*, May, vol. 1 Issue: 3, pp129–136

Mørkved, S. (2007) 'Pelvic floor muscle training during pregnancy and after delivery'. *Current Women's Health Reviews*, 3(1): 55–62

National Obesity Observatory (NOO) 'The economic burden of obesity', NHS, (2010)

'National trends in self-reported physical activity and sedentary behaviors among pregnant women' NHANES (1999–2006) *Preventative Medicine*, vol 50, issue 3, March 2010, pp123–128

Ned, Tijdschr Geneeskd (2005) 'Diabetes and pregnancy; the prevention of hypoglycaemia', Jan 22;149(4):172–6. [Article in Dutch] Visser GH, Evers IM, Kerssen A, de Valk HW

NICE Guidelines for Antenatal and Postnatal Mental Health, Guideline 45, April 2007

NICE (2008) *Guidelines for Antenatal Care*, March, Guideline 62

Owe, K., Mnystad, W., Bø K., (2009) 'Correlates of regular exercise during pregnancy: the Norwegian Mother and Child Cohort Study', *Scandinavian Journal of Medicine & Science in Sports*, October, 19 Issue number 5, p637–645

Parker, K.M., Smith, S.A., (2003) 'Aquatic Aerobic Exercise as a Means of Stress Reduction during Pregnancy', *Journal of Perinatal Education*, 12 (1):6-17

Price, S., (2007) *Mental Health in Pregnancy and Childbirth*, Churchill Livingstone/Elsevier

RCOG. (2006) Statement 4. Exercise in Pregnancy. www.rcog.org.uk [Accessed October 2012]

Sapsford, R.R., & Hodges, P.W., (2001) 'Contraction of the pelvic floor muscles during abdominal manouvers', *Archives of Physical Medicine and Rehabilitation*, vol 82: 1081–88

Sapsford, R.R., Hodges, P.W., Richardson, C.A., *et al*, (2001) 'Coactivation of the abdominal and pelvic floor muscles during voluntary exercises', *Neurourology and Urodynamics*, 20:31

Sattar, N. & Lean, M. (eds), (2007) *ABC of Obesity*, London: Blackwell Publishing

ScienceDaily. Retrieved March 20, 2013, from http://www.sciencedaily.com / releases/2011/04/110407101406.htm

Smith, S., Michel, Y., A, 'Pilot Study on the Effects of Aquatic Exercise and the Discomforts of Pregnancy' (2006) *Journal of Obstetric Gynaecological and Neonatal Nursing*, 35: 315–323

Sorenson, T.K., Williams, M.A., I-Min, L., (2003) 'Recreational physical activity during pregnancy and risk of preeclampsia' *Hypertension*, 41:273

ter Braak, E.W., Evers, I.M., Willem Erkelens, D, *et al.* (2002) 'Maternal hypoglycemia during pregnancy in type 1 diabetes: maternal and fetal consequences', *Diabetes Metab Res*, Rev. Mar–Apr; 18(2):96–105

Vallim, *et al.* (2011) 'Water exercises and quality of life during pregnancy', *Reproductive Health*, 8:14

Visser, G.H., Evers, I.M., Kerssen, A., *et al.* (2005) *Diabetes and Pregnancy; the prevention of hypoglycaemia*, Ned Tijdschr Geneeskd. Jan 22; 149(4)

Wahabi, H.A., Alzeidan, R.A. & Esmaeil, S.A., (2012) 'Pre-pregnancy care for women with pre-gestational diabetes mellitus: a systematic review and meta-analysis' *BMC Public Health*, 12:792

Waller, B.J., Johan, Daly D., (2009) 'Therapeutic aquatic exercise in the treatment of low back pain: a systematic review', *Clinical Rehabilitation*, January, vol. 23 Issue: Number 1 p3–14

Weston, C.F., O'Hare, J.P., Evans, J.M., *et al.* (1987) 'Hemodynamic changes in man during immersion in water at different temperatures', *Clin Sci*, 73 (6): 613-616)

Weir, Z., Bush, J., Robson, S.C., *et al.* (2010) 'Physical activity in pregnancy: a qualitative study of the beliefs of overweight and obese pregnant women BMC Pregnancy and Childbirth', 10:18 http://www.biomedcentral.com/1471-2393/10/18

INDEX